Undergraduate Medical Education and the Elective System

Undergraduate Medical Education and the Elective System:
Experience with the Duke Curriculum, 1966–75

Edited by
James F. Gifford, Jr.

Supervising editors
William G. Anlyan, M.D.
Ewald W. Busse, M.D.
Thomas D. Kinney, M.D.

Duke University Press   Durham, N.C.   1978

R.
747
D817
U53

Dedication

Thomas DeArman Kinney, M.D., Supervising Editor and a major contributor to this volume, died on June 12, 1977, as it was being prepared for publication. A graduate of the Duke University School of Medicine, Class of 1936, he returned to his alma mater in 1960 as Chairman of the Department of Pathology. He was a member of the original faculty group which conceived the new Duke curriculum in the 1960's. To its implementation and improvement he brought a wealth of experience gained at Johns Hopkins, Yale, Harvard, and Western Reserve. As Dean of Medical and Allied Health Education, he presided over its maturation. His contributions to this book made him its primary chronicler.

The editors and authors join in dedicating *Undergraduate Medical Education and the Elective System* to his memory.

Contents

Preface

The Flexner Report of 1910 climaxed more than half a century of efforts to improve the curricula of American medical schools and introduced an equally long era in which these curricula displayed marked uniformity. Two years of instruction in basic medical sciences, followed by two of clinical instruction in hospitals, became the accepted pedagogy for producing qualified practitioners, the initial governing assumption being the necessity of exposing students to the totality of biomedical knowledge. Although best remembered for its role in eliminating weak medical schools, the report was important also for helping to establish a normative educational model within which biomedical knowledge could be ordered and educational experimentation could take place. In the early 1950's, Western Reserve University demonstrated the viability of interdisciplinary approaches to teaching and, by so doing, led many schools to reexamine the effectiveness of their teaching methods. Later in the decade Stanford, Johns Hopkins, and several other schools experimented with variations in the sequence and time frame of medical education. Until the sixties, however, the four-year, two-part curriculum remained standard.

In the 1960's, however, a number of pressures combined to force many schools to reevaluate their curricula. Expansion of biomedical knowledge strained traditional courses beyond limits. Extension of postgraduate medical education, most often as preparation for specialization, raised questions about the proper scope of undergraduate medical education. The increasingly wide variety of careers open to medical graduates challenged the uniformity of course content and curricular structure. Demands by students as individuals for programs tailored to their individual abilities and goals were supported indirectly by competition for the best students from newly attractive programs in other scientific and technological fields. Social pressure mounted in favor of training more physicians from more diverse geographic, racial, and economic backgrounds.

The Duke University School of Medicine offered the first new model of medical education responsive to these pressures for change. Its first academic year included presentation by each basic science department of the core of principles and information deemed essential for any physician. In the second year students entered the wards of medicine, surgery, obstetrics and gynecology, pediatrics, and psychiatry as clinical clerks. The third and fourth years were given over to elective courses, equally divided between basic science and clinical subjects, chosen in accordance with the individual student's career goals with the guidance of an advisor from each of these general areas. A particular objective of the basic science program in the third year was to provide each student with opportunity to investigate a limited subject area in depth.

The purpose of this volume is to provide description and analysis of ten years of experience with this design. Beyond neatness, the ten-year demarcation is important for three reasons: (1) it represents the period during which a majority of the original planners of the new curriculum remained in leadership positions; (2) it is a period long enough to minimize the "Hawthorne effect," the effects of attitudes based primarily upon the experience of novelty; and (3) it permits longitudinal analysis of student attitudes toward their educational experience.

The chapters of this work were prepared independently, and are arranged in the following manner. The first chapter describes the historical background of the experiment, and particularly the circumstances unique to Duke. Chapter II summarizes the work of the Office of Admissions. The experience of each of the eight basic science departments and nine clinical departments is treated in single chapters. Special instructional programs, including those offering joint degrees, are reviewed in chapters XX to XXVI. The final chapters analyze the overall pattern of educational activity, student attitudes to their educational experiences, and the data presently available concerning graduates, concluding with a presentation of general conclusions and a look ahead.

As Dr. Jane Elchlepp points out in chapter XXVII, planning for the curriculum change described in this book took place during a period in which high national priority was placed upon biomedical research, implementation occurred during the era of emphasis upon medical manpower production, and currently the curriculum serves students and a society concerned about the adequacy of health care and health care delivery. The book itself is an interim report designed for comparison with reports of the many similar experiments made elsewhere, as preparation for responding still more creatively to the pressures and challenges of the years immediately ahead.

Acknowledgment

The contributors and editors acknowledge with thanks the funds provided by the National Library of Medicine, under grant number 1 RO1 LMO1778-01, for preparation and publication of this volume.

Alphabetical Listing of Contributors

(From Duke University unless otherwise indicated)

William G. Anlyan, M.D.   Vice President for Health Affairs; Professor of Surgery

William D. Bradford, M.D.   Associate Director for Undergraduate Medical Education; Associate Professor of Pathology; Assistant Professor of Pediatrics

Gert H. Brieger, M.D., PH.D.   Professor and Chairman, Department of History of Health Sciences, University of California, San Francisco.

Ewald W. Busse, M.D.   Associate Provost and Director of Medical and Allied Health Education; J. P. Gibbons Professor of Psychiatry

Arthur C. Chandler, Jr., M.D.   Associate Professor of Ophthalmology; Associate in Anatomy

Carl Eisdorfer, M.D., PH.D.   Professor and Chairman, Department of Psychiatry and Behavioral Sciences, University of Washington

Jane Elchlepp, M.D., PH.D.   Assistant Vice President for Health Affairs – Planning and Analysis; Associate Professor of Pathology

E. Harvey Estes, M.D.   Professor and Chairman, Community Health Sciences; Professor of Medicine

Johhnie L. Gallemore, M.D., J.D.   Associate Professor of Psychiatry – Duke; Associate Counsel (for Health), Interstate and Foreign Commerce Committee, U.S. House of Representatives

Samson R. Gross, PH.D.   Professor of Genetics and Biochemistry

Donald B. Hackel, M.D.   Professor of Pathology

Philip Handler, PH.D., D.SC., LITT.D., L.L.D., L.H.D.   James B. Duke Professor of Biochemistry, Duke; President, National Academy of Sciences, Washington, D.C.

Robert L. Hill, PH.D.   James B. Duke Professor and Chairman, Department of Biochemistry

Robert A. Jackson, M.A.   Research Assistant, Department of Sociology

Charles B. Johnson, ED.D.   Associate Registrar; Associate Director of Medical and Allied Health Education, Medical Education and Information Systems; Associate Professor of Education

Wolfgang K. Joklik, PH.D.   James B. Duke Professor and Chairman, Department of Microbiology and Immunology

Samuel L. Katz, M.D.   Wilburt C. Davison Professor and Chairman, Department of Pediatrics

Thomas D. Kinney, M.D.   Associate Provost and Director of Medical and Allied Health Education, Emeritus; Chairman, Department of Pathology, Emeritus; R. J. Reynolds Industries Professor of Medical Education; Professor of Pathology

Deborah W. Kredich, M.D.   Associate in Pediatrics

Nicholas M. Kredich, M.D.   Associate Professor of Medicine; Assistant Professor of Biochemistry

Richard G. Lester, M.D.   Professor and Chairman, Department of Radiology, University of Texas, Houston

Toshio Narahashi, PH.D.   Professor and Chairman, Department of Pharmacology, Northwestern University Medical School, Chicago

Suydam Osterhout, M.D., PH.D.   Associate Director of Medical and Allied Health Education, Medical School Admissions; Professor of Microbiology; Professor of Medicine

Roy T. Parker, M.D.   F. Bayard Carter Professor and Chairman, Department of Obstetrics and Gynecology

Eric Pfeiffer, M.D.   Professor of Psychiatry; Associate Director for Programs, Center for Studying Aging and Development

Theo C. Pilkington, PH.D.   Professor and Chairman of Biomedical Engineering; Professor of Electrical Engineering

Jack J. Preiss, PH.D.   Professor of Sociology

J. David Robertson, M.D., PH.D.   James B. Duke Professor and Chairman, Department of Anatomy

Wendell F. Rosse, M.D.   Professor of Medicine; Associate Professor of Immunology

David C. Sabiston, Jr., M.D.   James B. Duke Professor and Chairman, Department of Surgery

Eugene A. Stead, Jr., M.D.   Florence McAlister Professor of Medicine

Daniel C. Tosteson, M.D.   Dean of the Faculty and Carolina Shields Walker Professor of Physiology, Harvard Medical School, Cambridge, Mass.

James B. Wyngaarden, M.D.   Frederic M. Hanes Professor and Chairman, Department of Medicine

History and Admissions

I. Historical Background

Philip Handler, PH.D.

Eugene A. Stead, Jr., M.D.

The curriculum introduced in 1930 by the originating faculty of the Duke University School of Medicine was a model of flexibility within tradition. The tradition of a four-year medical curriculum, with the first two years devoted to instruction in the basic sciences and the last two to clinical clerkships, had been established at The Johns Hopkins University School of Medicine and made normative for American medical education by the influence of Abraham Flexner's *Medical Education in the United States and Canada.* Since a majority of its first faculty were recruited from the staff of the Hopkins, this tradition provided Duke with a working philosophy and with a pattern for organizing the day-to-day operations of the medical school and hospital.

Flexibility within this tradition, for faculty and students alike, was to be safeguarded by utilizing only 54 percent of the clock hours of the curriculum for required courses. The remainder of the hours were to be devoted to elective courses through which a student might prepare himself either for general practice, by spreading his elective choices widely through the curriculum, or for specialty practice, by concentrating them in one department.[1]

The pressures on this curriculum design, however, proved overwhelming, particularly as advances in biomedical knowledge transformed the content of most of the traditional courses and as greater emphasis was placed upon broad understanding of the patient in his social environment. Each new discovery or improvement in technique in every field forced reconsideration of the design of required courses. Allowance of more required time to any one department brought parallel demands from others. The offering of many electives to small groups of students was expensive in terms of faculty time. Accordingly, almost every academic year witnessed a decrease in the percentage of elective hours in the curriculum design (Table I – I). In 1955 a site visitor from the Commonwealth Fund commented that nearly everyone he saw exhibited a real interest in the educational aspect of his work but noted that the "whole four-year program amounts to 5,148 teaching hours of which only 17 are free time. This is really tight!"[2]

Table I–1. Teaching hours assigned to required courses and free time, selected years, 1930–65.[3]

Year	Percentage of teaching hours assigned to required courses	Percentage of teaching hours assigned to electives and free time
1930	54	46
1935	72	28
1940	83	17
1945	92	8
1950	97	3
1955	97	3
1960	84	16

In the years following 1955 the pressure on the curriculum was eased on paper by increasing the number of clock hours presupposed for the entire curriculum, as stated in the catalogue. This was at best, however, a temporary solution to an enduring problem. During the academic year 1955–56 the medical school faculty spent considerable time "taking stock," as they put it, of medical education generally. Among the specific proposals for improvement of the curriculum which emerged from these discussions was one by Dr. Philip Handler, then Professor of Biochemistry, for a training program for clinical investigators.

Handler came to Duke in 1939, fresh from his doctoral studies at Illinois. His rise to the position of Chairman of the Department of Biochemistry occurred during the time that the teaching of biochemistry assumed a more and more important role in the curricula of American medical schools. By 1955 he recognized that, although the availability of funds had made possible a significant increase in the quantity of medical research following World War II, medical curricula generally had not made specific provision for the training of students both as investigators and as clinicians. He saw particular need to train students who, at some future date, would become members of the basic science faculties of medical schools.

Handler projected, for a small number of superior students, an intensive training period of nine months which students could enter at any time after completion of the first two years of medical school. The heart of the program was a central teaching facility, where students familarized themselves with advanced research tools in a variety of fields by proceeding through a series of experiments under the guidance of specialists. This first phase lasted for sixteen weeks. During the following twenty weeks, each student was required to design and undertake a small research project of his own, preferably one involving more than one traditional discipline. Accompanying this laboratory experience were two series of seminar meetings, one stressing the experimental bases for theories current in the preclinical sciences and the other providing a grounding in such areas as mathematics, statistics, electronics, and instrumentation.

Handler hoped that out of each class of eighteen students as many as five or six would complete requirements for the Ph.D. before resuming their medical education. At the end of their internships and residencies they would be well suited, by the variety and interdisciplinary nature of their education, for teaching or research in either clinical medicine or preclinical science.[4]

Handler's proposal won the endorsement of the Duke faculty. The chairmen of the departments of medicine and surgery, Drs. J. Deryl Hart and Eugene A. Stead, Jr. respectively, agreed that a student could spend one quarter in the program in substitution for one of the two required quarters in each of medicine and surgery. This decision made it possible for the student to elect what finally was called the Research Training Program and, by attending school for two summers, to graduate on schedule with his medical school class.

Stead was particularly enthusiastic. He believed firmly that the establishment of patterns of thinking, of curiosity, and of satisfaction which would lead a student to continue his education beyond medical school was the proper primary goal of the undergraduate medical curriculum, and that this goal was best accomplished by placing the students in contact with young teachers sensitive to the human needs of their patients. Convinced that the large majority of medical students possessed outstanding abilities, he favored experiments which would fit medical education to the individual aspirations of each student. As a clinical chief he sought similarly broad experiences for his staff—for example, by making departmental funds available to staff members so that they might gain the benefits of psychoanalysis.

Aided by support from Duke University, The Commonwealth Fund and The National Institute of Health, the Research Training Program was initiated in the fall of 1959. Within two years, sixteen medical schools sent visitors to observe the program and over one hundred additional written requests for information on the program were received.[5] Under the direction of Dr. James B. Wyngaarden, Associate Professor of Medicine and Biochemistry, the program quickly came to serve not only undergraduate medical students but also graduates of medical schools who desired a year of research training as part of their post-doctoral work. Within Duke University, the program became an important bridge between the medical school faculty and University science departments.

The only criticism after two years of the program came from some of the undergraduate medical students it was originally intended to serve. These students were ambivalent about spending a year in research before having had opportunity for clinical experience with patients. Years of anticipation of patient contact made them reluctant to interrupt their progress toward this goal. By 1961, Handler and Wyngaarden began to think about allowing entrance into the Research Training Program after the third year of medical school in order to satisfy this desire.

The Research Training Program experiment coincided with years of transition at the Duke University Medical Center. The post-war growth of both the

Medical School and the Hospital necessitated extensive planning for future plant development. Technical questions, such as whether to add to existing buildings or build new ones, could not be answered adequately apart from reconsideration of the objectives and philosophy of the medical school faculty. With the support of The Duke Endowment, the management consultant firm of Booz, Allen and Hamilton was engaged to facilitate this planning. Their report, delivered to the Medical School and the University as of August 11, 1961, stressed, among other elements, the necessity of strong basic science departments for a medical school of national reputation. Department chairmen were encouraged to reflect upon how to strengthen their programs.

The years 1959 to 1961 also brought the retirements of Dr. Wilbert C. Davison, Duke's first dean, and of several of the original department chairmen. Change for the future was facilitated by this circumstance. Dr. Barnes Woodhall, who had emphasized the need for the Booz, Allen and Hamilton study, succeeded Davison as dean in 1960 and would lead in implementing its recommendations. Meanwhile Dr. Hart, who retired as Professor of Surgery to become President of Duke University, brought into being closer working relationships between the Medical School and the University, patterns that continued under his successors.

In this atmosphere, in November of 1961, a group of department chairmen in the Medical School held a meeting in Dr. Handler's office, the original purpose of which none can recall. Present, in addition to Handler, were Stead, Dr. Thomas D. Kinney, Chairman of Pathology, and Dr. Jerome S. Harris, Chairman of Pediatrics. Concluding their formal business quickly, they turned their conversation to the enduring problem of the curriculum.

Points of agreement quickly appeared. The curriculum clearly was too rigid to allow students to vary their preparation for the variety of careers available to individuals holding the M.D., and there was no opportunity for the student to learn one field in depth. The group was concerned about the fact that most medical students lived through the first two years of the curriculum in frustration. Their image of a physician had been framed by early contact with their family doctors and they arrived expecting to learn to behave as physicians immediately. For them the basic medical sciences seemed less a preparation for clinical education and more a series of hurdles to be overcome on their way to that education.

According to this argument it was only years later, after the students experienced both the joys and the frustrations of clinical practice and fully realized the limitations of current techniques, that they recognized the importance of the material they once committed to rote memory in basic science courses but had long since forgotten. By then, however, the demands of practice, of family, of finances, or other impediments usually precluded any return to scientific study.

The Western Reserve School of Medicine had attempted to alleviate some of these problems by abandoning all thought of total coverage in any given preclinical course in order to place emphasis, by using interdisciplinary teaching methods, upon the mechanisms of disease. Emphasis also was placed upon the cultivation of habits of self-education. Kinney had been at Western Reserve as a professor of pathology, the position at the interface of basic science and clinical medicine in the traditional curriculum. Granted the importance of an interdisciplinary perspective for the practice of modern medicine, he argued, the fault of the Western Reserve system in practice had been that most students were not adequately familiar with the language of medicine used in the interdisciplinary courses and, therefore, that some core material in traditional fields was necessary prior to integrated teaching. At once idealist and pragmatist, Stead supported the need for the student to know the language necessary to the understanding of medical science. Mastery of the language, in his opinion, should be the primary qualification for entry into medical school.

Given the tradition of departmental autonomy at Duke, any curriculum change would have to be approved by the department chairmen. Harris strongly emphasized this requirement. Biochemist as well as pediatrician, he, like Stead, defined medicine broadly. The domains of the department as expressed in the allocation of required teaching time, he recognized, would have to be cut down considerably if meaningful change was to occur. Powerful resistance could be expected.

Another feature of the discussion was the regret that the sequential nature of the current curriculum sometimes necessitated deferral of a career decision with respect to the subsequent specialty training until late in the fourth year of medical school. It was agreed that some other arrangement might permit more students to make earlier career decisions so that at least the fourth year, and perhaps the third, could be constructed in accord with the future goals of the individual student.

The group began to consider the possibility of a new curriculum in which as much as possible of the heart of the first two years of the old curriculum was offered to students in a single first year, which would focus upon the basic principles of each of the basic medical sciences. Each of the clinical departments then would present an abbreviated clinical rotation to the students in the second year, each department determining for itself the mix of didactic instruction and ward or outpatient clinic experience it would present to the neophyte physicians. They then would return to the study in depth of one or more areas of basic medical science in the third year, and in the fourth year would select clinical electives correlated with their career goals.

The excitement of this discussion was quickly shared with others. Among the first to add their viewpoints was Dr. Daniel C. Tosteson, newly elected chairman of the Department of Physiology. Tosteson was adamant that all notions of devising a new curriculum for some students while retaining the traditional structure for others be abandoned. When he won this point, the essence of a new curriculum philosophy existed. Handler reported their conversations to Dean Woodhall and asked that he, Stead, Kinney, Harris and Tosteson be appointed as an ad hoc committee of the medical faculty to bring the proposal to the entire faculty. Woodhall made the necessary appointments on December 6, 1961.[6]

Handler spent his Christmas vacation drafting a proposal for the committee to consider.[7] The committee hoped that the entire process of translating the general concepts into a specific reality might be finished by the fall of 1964 and the new curriculum initiated at that time, but it was to take two additional years. During 1962 the ad hoc committee served as the focus for a series of discussions between themselves and other members of the faculty in which the major problems of philosophy and practice were addressed. Two ideas won ready acceptance; that students should have multiple paths through the curriculum to permit them to pursue their individual interests and that admission to Duke should not be entirely restricted to students with strong backgrounds in science. Other problems, however, proved less tractable.

The most obvious task was to be certain that each of the departments responsible for instruction in the first year would not overburden the students by putting all materials formerly taught under the old structure into the new core courses. Preclinical faculty had to be convinced that although in their first exposure all students would be taught somewhat less material than previously, the opportunity would come later to teach a great deal more to some students. Also, each department would have to be more aware of what the others were doing so as to eliminate as much redundancy in presentations to students as possible. The burden of change under the proposed structure fell more heavily on the preclinical departments. Instruction in the second year, by the clinical departments, would continue to be by clinical clerkship. This disparity between what the new curriculum asked of basic science and of clinical faculty did not seem totally in the spirit of the new curriculum, but could not be entirely eliminated.

Other problems affected the third and fourth years, particularly since no specific plans for the fourth year had been developed. The easiest arrangement for the third year appeared to be for medical students to return to specific basic science departments and there be treated as graduate students. This created the temptation, however, to regard the third year simply as opportunity to teach everything which had to be omitted from the first year. This temptation was particularly strong for the Department of Anatomy. Under the traditional concept, Anatomy had always been assigned a large share of the first year; therefore, they lost more clock hours than any other department under the reorganization. All departments, however, experienced serious difficulty in redefining their objectives in specific terms to meet the goals of the third and fourth years.

As the sense of difficulty mounted, resistance grew within the faculty. By December of 1962, at least some members of most departments viewed the third year primarily as the opportunity for formal instruction, with elective opportunity only for the gifted and venturesome. This seemed to reintroduce the idea, long before rejected, that two curricula would coexist at Duke.

"Slowly," Handler lamented, "I come round to believing that if we cannot convert the curriculum over—whole hog—to the kind of experience we originally discussed, I think we will have spun our wheels vigorously but to no useful end." [8]

In this mood, on January 11, 1963, Handler proposed to the ad hoc committee that the third year should offer students a choice from among a series of multidisciplinary, cooperative teaching and learning experiences for which the current Research Training Program would serve as a model. Programs devoted to such areas as neurobiology, neoplasia, genetics and metabolism, psychobiology or the cardiovascular system would enliven the curriculum by permitting the student to study in depth in one field while emphasizing the continuity between clinical experience and study of basic science generally. Fourth-year courses might well follow a similar model, emphasizing the clinical aspects of the areas of concentration. This idea broke the bottleneck: by providing a model within which to consider new offerings, it changed the question being asked by the Duke faculty from whether a new curriculum could be initiated to how best to do it.

In the spring of 1963 a revised version of the original plan was circulated among the faculty by the ad hoc committee and discussed at the first of a series of faculty retreats. To make the curriculum as flexible as possible, this draft suggested, the student should be free to arrange his work in the third and fourth years in any sequence of clinical and preclinical experiences he chose, thus potentially making those years a single integrated learning experience if he so desired. Whenever chosen, third-year content might involve concentration in one or more basic science departmental electives, participation in the Research Training Program, or enrollment in a basic science graduate program. In the fourth year, this draft strongly suggested, the student should take care not to choose work in the field of his intended internship; rather, he should elect work in complementary areas. At the very least, experience in two clinical fields was required. Close contact between students and faculty advisors was considered essential to the success of the proposal, yet responsibility for the integration of medical knowledge rested with the individual students. [9]

With the publication of this revised plan the ad hoc committee ceased to exist. Its formal successor, a Committee on the Curriculum chaired by Professor of Medicine Herbert O. Sieker, was already at work. This committee, from late 1962 onward, coordinated departmental plans for curriculum revision through two subcommittees, one concerned with the first and third (basic science) years and one with the second and fourth (clinical) years. Later separate committees were formed for each of the four years. Dr. Woodhall and the Associate Dean of Medicine, Dr. William G. Anlyan, convened periodic faculty retreats involving twenty-five or more members, away from the University, where successive drafts of the overall proposal were hammered out and agreed to. The result of the work of these groups, the new curriculum structure itself, is shown in Table I – 2 and described in detail in subsequent chapters. Attention must be given here, however, to the related tasks of seeking outside criticism of, and financial support for, the new proposal.

Professional meetings, beginning in the fall of 1963, provided the primary means of soliciting both. Conscious from the beginning that the elective curriculum was experimental, the Duke faculty shared drafts of their proposal with interested friends and solicited information on proposed changes elsewhere. Since the frustrations felt at Duke with the traditional curriculum were common at other medical schools as well, the proposal generated considerable discussion. One enthusiastic reader asked for permission to publish details of the plan, even though it was still in tentative form, because he regarded it as "the second Flexner report." [10] As interest began to build, Dr. Anlyan, who in 1964 had become Dean of the School of Medicine, approached J. Quigg Newton, President of the Commonwealth Fund, to ask if The Fund might consider support of the new proposal. The Duke faculty hoped that such a grant would, beyond its immediate value, stimulate additional support from other sources.

Although the major support for the elective curriculum came from the continuing contributions of Duke University and The Duke Endowment, new funds for support of additional faculty in the basic sciences were critical to its success. The total amount needed for nine positions during the first five and one half years of operation was $750,000. Early in the fall of 1964 Dr. Anlyan requested this amount from the Commonwealth Fund. Its staff immediately sent the curriculum proposal to several medical reviewers, thereby enlarging discussion of the elective curriculum among medical educators.

The reports from the reviewers and from other medical educators encountered at conventions were favorable. High regard for the Duke faculty, and particularly for those whose names were associated with the origins and development of the proposal, figured prominently in the responses. Perhaps even more important was the general recognition that the elective curriculum was a radically experimental approach to problems long recognized, but not effectively addressed, by medical educators. The national implications of the experiment were recognized almost before it began. As a reason for support, most cited the need for multiple pathways through the curriculum to meet varied career goals. Finally, even those who were unwilling to concede that the proposed changes were radical suggested that the faculty would of necessity devote more time and attention to the business of education, and thus in the long run do a better job with the students. [11]

The staff of The Commonwealth Fund paid particular attention to a critique written by Dr. Joseph T. Wearn, Emeritus Dean of the Western Reserve University School of Medicine. Wearn had coordinated the efforts of that faculty to reorganize basic science instruction at Western Reserve on

Table I-2. Structure of the Duke Curriculum

Year	1	2	3	4
Traditional curriculum 1930–1965	Basic Science	Basic Science	Clinical Science	Clinical Science
Elective curriculum 1966–	Basic Science Core	Clinical Science Core	Basic Science Electives	Clinical Science Electives
Content of elective curriculum	*Term 1* Anatomy Biochemistry Physiology Neurological sciences Genetics — Introduction to Clinical medicine / *Term 2* Pathology Microbiology Pharmacology Human Behavior	Medicine Surgery Obstetrics Pediatrics Psychiatry	Elective courses in all departments	

an interdisciplinary basis a decade earlier. He raised several issues, the most important of which was that the staff of The Commonwealth Fund satisfy itself that thorough planning had preceded the proposal. He cautioned that many unanticipated problems would inevitably tax the creativity of the Duke faculty. He questioned the assumption that the curriculum would allow for early career decisions, suggesting that many medical students changed their minds repeatedly, and wondered if the new curriculum made provision for this. Similarly, he asked if the Duke proposal gave adequate recognition to the need for continuity in learning about the patient, his illnesses, and his health between illnesses, since a majority of students would go into some form of practice. Some students, he argued, might need to be broadly prepared to take direct care of the sick. He supported funding of the proposal provided these questions, especially the one on the adequacy of planning, were answered, and applauded the clearly experimental nature of the plan.[12]

Site visitors from The Commonwealth Fund presented these questions, along with many others, to the Duke faculty in December, 1964. The visitors were quickly satisfied concerning the adequacy of the planning process, which had included trial introductions of the elective curriculum structure in the departments of pathology and physiology. Handler pointed out to them that no one was sure how students selected their career fields and that in fact some students adhered to decisions made before entering medical school while others repeatedly changed their minds. He argued that presentation of the wide variety of career possibilities early in the medical school experience should aid at least a minority in coming more quickly to a meaningful and firm choice. Also, the option to choose a broad rather than a concentrated range of experience over the last two years would provide another appropriate opportunity for the undecided to make meaningful choices. Since a survey of students in two consecutive classes indicated that at least four of every five students under the traditional curriculum were making what they felt were career choices by the end of the second year, the primary emphasis would be upon providing a better basis for decision-making.

Given the increasing importance of scientific research in modern medical practice, the specialization of the Duke faculty, and the fact that virtually no Duke graduates were entering general practice, the elective curriculum was not specifically directed to the production of family practitioners. Stead particularly felt that the solo practitioner was gradually being replaced by more specialized physicians associated in group practices, and it was this role that the faculty anticipated many of its graduates would fill. Many of the faculty argued that although the students would experience continuity in patient care at different times and in different ways depending on their interests, there was no reason why this experience could not adequately be included in a wide variety of curriculum sequences. Convinced that the entire Duke faculty supported Stead's position that the essential problem of curriculum was to focus upon teaching students how to learn and enjoy learning, one site visitor reported that "this program is so excellent that it is difficult to describe it other than in superlatives, but I shall try to restrain the wild use of these as much as possible." [13]

Upon the enthusiastic recommendation of its staff, the Board of Directors of the Commonwealth Fund voted, in February, 1965, to provide the full $750,000.00 to finance the additional faculty members needed to permit the inauguration of the elective curriculum, [14] which then was announced for the fall of 1966. Its aims were: "(1) to provide a strong academic basis for a lifetime of growth within the profession of medicine, with the development of technical competency, proficiency, and the proper attitudes peculiar to the practice of medicine as well as appreciation of of the broader social and service responsibilities; (2) to establish for the first year a basic science program which will fulfill the purposes of the increasingly heterogeneous student body; (3) to offer both clinical and basic science education simultaneously; (4) to permit the student to explore his personal intellectual preferences and capabilities; (5) to allow study in depth in selected areas, either basic science or clinical; (6) to provide greater freedom of course selection, and thus to encourage earlier career decision; (7) to achieve better integration of the medical school curriculum with residency training and the practice of medicine." [15]

Only a history of the attainments of Duke graduates, decades from now, will permit final comment on the first and most important goal. The chapters which follow present a preliminary description and analysis of the elective curriculum in terms of the other six goals.

References

1. W. C. Davison, "Liberalizing the Curriculum." *Southern Medical Journal* 21 (Dec., 1928): 983–87. See also Davison, "An M.D. Degree Five Years after High School." *J.A.M.A.* 90 (2 June, 1928): 1812–16, and Davison, "The Duke University School of Medicine." *Transactions of the Medical Society of the State of North Carolina* 74 (1927): 35–39.
2. Charles O. Warren, M.D., Memorandum. "Duke University School of Medicine, Durham, North Carolina," Sept. 15, 1955. In Commonwealth Fund Papers.
3. Statistics in this table are prepared from information contained in successive issues of the *Bulletin* of the Duke University School of Medicine.
4. Philip Handler, M.D., to Lester J. Evans, M.D., Dec. 26, 1957. In Commonwealth Fund Papers.
5. James B. Wyngaarden, M.D., to Roderick Heffron, M.D., Nov. 30, 1961. Letter and enclosures in Commonwealth Fund Papers.
6. Barnes Woodhall, M.D., to Philip Handler, M.D., Dec. 6, 1961. In Philip Handler Papers.
7. "A New Curriculum in the Duke University School of Medicine." Undated. In Philip Handler Papers.
8. Philip Handler, M.D., to Drs. Kenney, Tosteson, Harris, and Stead, Dec. 6, 1962. Copy in Philip Handler Papers.

9. "A New Curriculum in the School of Medicine, Duke University (Revised Plan)." March, 1963. In Philip Handler Papers.

10. Charles G. Child, III, M.D., to William G. Anlyan, M.D., Nov. 13, 1964. Copy in Thomas D. Kinney Papers.

11. Robert J. Glaser, M.D., to J. Quigg Newton, Sept. 23, 1964; L. T. Coggeshall, M.D., to Roderick Heffron, M.D., Oct. 2, 1964; W. Barry Wood, Jr., M.D., to Roderick Heffron, M.D., Sept. 30, 1964. In Commonwealth Fund Papers.

12. Joseph T. Wearn, M.D., to Dr. Roderick Heffron, Oct. 17, 1964. In Commonwealth Fund Papers.

13. Memorandum, "Duke University School of Medicine." Dec. 15, 1964. By Roderick Heffron, M.D. In Commonwealth Fund Papers.

14. Memorandum, "Duke University Medical School, New Curriculum." Feb. 25, 1965. In Commonwealth Fund Papers.

15. Duke Medical School *Bulletin*, 1966, pp. 4–5.

II. The Elective Curriculum and the Admissions Committee

Suydam Osterhout, M.D., PH.D.*

Introduction

Each student who intends medicine as a career must make two decisions: the choice of schools to which to apply and the choice of which offer of entrance to accept. These decisions are influenced by such variables as the reputation of each medical school, its geographic location, its premedical requirements, the number of applicants relative to the number of places, the legal residence of the student and his family, the health and income of the family, parental attitudes and alumni status, the age and marital status of the applicant, and finally, the number of acceptances that the student holds. In this list also should be mentioned the curriculum of each medical school.

For some students, pressure to gain admittance to any medical school precludes consideration of other questions, while for others the curricular contents of a medical school are not of great importance so long as "you make me a doctor like uncle Joe." For the more discerning student, however, curricular considerations stimulate the imagination, suggest the future, and may become a significant factor in making the second decision. The purpose of this chapter is to explore the effects of the newly instituted elective curriculum on the activities of the Admissions Committee, while recognizing that the complexities of the admissions process preclude isolation of the effects of any single variable.

Sources of information valued by students prior to entering medical school

Medical students who enrolled at Duke under both the traditional and elective curricula reported reliance upon similar sources of information in following their impressions of what medical school would be like. First in importance to the two groups were the opinions of students already in

*The author wishes to acknowledge gratefully the work of May G. King, Administrative Assistant for Medical School Admissions, in the preparation of the tables.

medical schools, whether at Duke or elsewhere, closely followed by those of physicians who were family friends or family members. Secondary importance was attached to information from medical school publications and from college and medical school faculty. Other sources were important only in isolated instances. A summary of the data from which these conclusions are drawn appears in Table II–1.

Table II–1. Importance of sources of information concerning medical school to students prior to enrollment (first figures are percentages, those in parentheses are number of students)

	Traditional curriculum (N=235: classes entering 1961–63)				
	Very important	Fairly important	Of minor importance	Not at all important	No answer
Medical school bulletins	7.2 (17)	37.4 (88)	36.2 (85)	15.7 (37)	3.4 (8)
Medical students at Duke	37.4 (88)	28.9 (68)	13.2 (31)	17.9 (42)	2.6 (6)
Medical students at other schools	29.4 (69)	32.3 (76)	20.9 (49)	14.5 (34)	3.0 (7)
Family members who are doctors	20.9 (49)	12.3 (29)	7.2 (17)	51.9 (122)	7.7 (18)
Family physician	15.3 (36)	26.8 (63)	28.9 (68)	23.8 (56)	5.1 (12)
Physicians who are friends	26.0 (61)	31.5 (74)	25.1 (59)	14.0 (33)	3.4 (8)
Medical school faculty	18.7 (44)	29.8 (70)	29.8 (70)	15.3 (36)	6.4 (15)
College faculty	11.5 (27)	23.0 (54)	31.9 (75)	27.2 (64)	6.4 (15)
Books, movies, plays	2.1 (5)	6.4 (15)	14.5 (34)	27.7 (65)	49.4 (116)
Other	6.4 (15)	2.6 (6)	0.4 (1)	10.2 (24)	80.4 (189)
	Elective curriculum (N=254: classes entering 1966–68)				
	Very important	Fairly important	Of minor importance	Not at all important	No answer
Medical school bulletins	9.8 (25)	37.0 (94)	40.9 (104)	9.4) (24)	2.8 (7)
Medical students at Duke	28.7 (73)	29.9 (76)	16.5 (42)	20.5 (52)	4.3 (11)
Medical students at other schools	31.1 (79)	38.6 (98)	20.0 (51)	8.7 (22)	1.6 (4)
Family members who are doctors	20.1 (51)	9.8 (25)	8.7 (22)	55.9 (142)	5.5 (14)
Family physician	11.0 (28)	18.9 (48)	30.3 (77)	34.6 (88)	5.1 (13)
Physicians who are friends	26.0 (66)	33.1 (84)	20.9 (53)	16.5 (42)	3.5 (9)
Medical School faculty	19.3 (49)	26.8 (68)	27.6 (70)	22.8 (58)	3.5 (9)
College faculty	4.7 (12)	24.4 (62)	40.2 (102)	24.0 (61)	6.7 (14)
Books, movies, plays	2.0 (5)	9.4 (24)	19.3 (49)	31.9 (81)	37.4 (95)
Other	10.2 (26)	5.1 (13)	0.8 (2)	11.4 (29)	72.4 (184)

*Data for this table collected and compiled by Dr. Jack J. Preiss, Department of Sociology, Duke University.

The applicant pool

The decision of the medical school admissions committee on each application is influenced by a large number of variables. First, and most important, is the size and quality of applicant pool. Between 1966 and 1974 the number of students applying to medical schools increased markedly both nationally and locally, as did the number of applications filed by each applicant. The rate of increase was greater at Duke than nationwide. Over the past three years, the average score by Duke students on the MCAT also has risen appreciably compared to the national norm. A summary of this experience is provided in Table II–2.

Table II–2. Application experience of Admissions Committee, Duke University School of Medicine, 1963–74*

Enter-ing class	Total national applic.	Total Duke applic.	Inter-viewed locally	Inter-viewed regionally	Inter-viewed on trip	Class size	Duke enter MCAT	National enter MCAT
1963	17,668	1,156	–	–	–	82	581	546
1964	19,168	1,072	–	–	–	82	594	556
1965	18,703	1,118	–	–	–	80	577	558
1966	18,250	1,225	296	336	206	81	601	560
1967	18,724	1,347	280	400	188	86	618	570
1968	21,118	1,436	303	556	181	86	614	576
1969	24,465	1,685	328	582	194	86	631	578
1970	24,987	1,804	369	569	240	104	609	571
1971	29,172	2,150	491	708	246	105	599	572
1972	36,135	3,151	546	759	370	114	612	543
1973	40,506	3,621	551	960	501	114	625	548
1974	42,624	3,935	610	952	547	115	618	550

*AAMC estimates

Three new variables influenced the size and configuration of the applicant pool at Duke during the period when the new curriculum was introduced. The first involved the institution of new programs: a Medical Scientist Training Program for twelve students in each entering class, combined M.D. – Ph.D. programs in Biomedical Engineering and in Medical History, a combined M.D. – J.D. Program, and M.D. – M.P.H. Program. Each of these is described in detail elsewhere in this volume.

Table II–3. Application experience with black students, Duke University School of Medicine, 1969–75.

	1969	1970	1971	1972	1973	1974	1975
Number of black applicants	23	47	68	134	123	145	161
Black applicants accepted	7	12	13	12	15	20	22
Black females accepted	4	3	4	0	2	10	6
Black females enrolled	1	1	3	0	0	3	4
Black males accepted	3	9	9	12	13	10	16
Black males enrolled	1	6	5	6	6	6	8
Black applicants enrolled	2	7	8	6	6	9	11

Table II–4. Application experience with North Carolina students, Duke University School of Medicine, 1963–75

	1963	1964	1965	1966	1967	1968	1969	1970	1971	1972	1973	1974	1975
Total applications received:	805	1131	1118	1225	1347	1436	1685	1804	2150	3151	3621	3935	4242
North Carolina applications received:	79	*	*	73	65	85	111	129	180	249	243	307	316
North Carolina accepted applicants:	24	*	18	17	13	26	22	46	42	49	44	52	41
North Carolina enrolled students:	15	17	8	8	6	15	10	25	26	30	28	36	32

*Data unavailable.

Table II–5. Application experience with female students, Duke University School of Medicine, 1965–75

	1965	1966	1967	1968	1969	1970	1971	1972	1973	1974	1975
Total number applications:	55	85	120	129	132	171	267	455	638	815	864
Total number accepted:	13	14	20	14	14	27	30	50	60	73	70
Total number enrolled:	7	8	10	8	3	8	14	18	32	31	34

The second variable involved parallel efforts to enlarge the representation of black students, North Carolinians, and women in each entering class. The effort to increase North Carolina enrollment was supported in part by the decision of the North Carolina General Assembly to provide capitation grants with partial tuition remission for needy students from the state. Experience with the influence of these variables is presented in Tables II–3 through II–5.

The third variable was that, beginning in 1966, a concerted effort was made to recruit students at schools with reputations for high academic standards. Starting with four trips involving two members to the Admissions Committee on each trip, approximately one week is spent visiting two or three schools and interviewing applicants interested in our School of Medicine. Interview notes so created are forwarded back to the Medical School Admission Office for incorporation into the applicant's file, following which the applicant is reviewed in depth by three members of the committee. For the past three years a fifth recruiting trip has been made by two women members of the Medical School Admissions Committee to schools whose student body is made up predominately of women. A comparison of applications received from the target schools is presented in Table II–6.

Table II–6. Duke University School of Medicine applicants from Northeastern schools recruited by Admissions Committee during two five-year periods

School	1961	1962	1963	1964	1965	1971	1972	1973	1974	1975
Amherst	5	–	–	5	5	16	11	22	25	30
Brown	–	–	6	8	9	22	28	36	58	52
Columbia-Barnard	5	9	10	18	15	51	56	78	102	81
Dartmouth	15	10	7	17	23	25	38	53	57	56
Harvard-Radcliffe	14	10	21	28	31	79	101	128	132	140
M. I. T.	–	–	8	8	–	28	59	56	48	70
Mt. Holyoke	–	–	–	–	–	5	6	10	15	18
Princeton	17	15	22	15	27	38	37	68	77	95
Smith	–	–	–	–	–	8	10	22	30	15
University of Pennsylvania	8	8	13	24	18	33	59	66	65	66
Wellesley	–	–	–	–	–	5	14	19	19	29
Wesleyan	–	–	8	10	6	–	12	16	13	12
Williams	–	–	–	5	8	2 1	16	20	30	31
Yale	9	12	12	23	20	41	81	94	115	105
Total	73	64	107	161	162	372	518	688	786	800

The committee function

The Admissions Committee begins its work each year with an August 1 mailing of application materials to applicants on an accumulated mailing list. Completed applications are continuously received until December 1. Each application is first screened by the Chairman of the Admissions Committee to determine if the applicant is competitive. Non-competitive applicants are informed as quickly as possible; marginal applications are held for such additional information as recommendations, repeat Medical College Admissions Test (MCAT) scores, or first semester grades.

An interview is required of the candidate who is competitive. If the student attends an undergraduate college within a 300-mile radius of Durham, North Carolina, he or she is invited to the Medical Center. Whenever possible, the individual interview committee will be composed of a basic science faculty member, a clinical faculty member, and the Chairman of the Admissions Committee. Such committees meet three times weekly from late September through February, interviewing eight or nine students per day for twenty to thirty minutes each.

After an interview is completed, each member of the interview committee is asked to rate the applicant on a sliding numerical scale. Specific criteria considered include overall academic achievement, academic achievement in the sciences, academic improvement, school attended, letters of recommendation from faculty, Medical College Admission Test scores, participation in extracurricular activities, knowledge of the demands of medicine and the ability to communicate. Essential qualifications for admission also include favorable assessment of the applicant's character, integrity, intelligence, study habits, and motivation. The numerical evaluations of the committee members are averaged.

Students who attend undergraduate colleges beyond the 300-mile radius are interviewed by Regional Representatives (graduates of the Duke University School of Medicine in practice in this country, Europe, or Asia). These representatives forward a report of the interview to the Admissions Office. Additionally, five times each year the committee sends two members to the Northeast to visit schools with reputations for high academic standards to interview prospective applicants. Interview notes are similarly forwarded to the Admissions Office. In either case, a screening process is conducted by three members of the Admissions Committee just as in the case of applicants seen locally. Numerical evaluations are assigned and averaged.

Applicants with the highest numerical ratings are presented to the full Admissions Committee at evening meetings held approximately ten times a year. Presently this committee stands at approximately twenty members; the chairman, his administrative assistant, whenever possible a faculty representative from each department of the Medical School, and two medical students. A member of the interview committee who voted on an individual application presents that candidate to the full committee for consideration.

Applicants approved for admission by the full committee are sent letters of acceptance in order of the excellence of their qualifications. Enclosed, if requested on the original application, is an application for financial assistance. These are processed, as quickly as possible, by a Financial Aid Committee, and each applicant is notified as to what assistance he or she may expect from Duke. Applicants then decide whether or not to accept the offer of acceptance.

The bulk of acceptance activity is completed by December, although it continues into March. In April the strongest applicants who have been voted acceptable by the full Admissions Committee, but who have not been sent letters of acceptance because of limitations of space, are offered a place on the alternate list. Once this list is complete, all remaining applicants are informed that they will not be offered a place in the entering class.

Children of Medical School alumni are given special consideration in that regardless of the credentials presented, the student is interviewed. In addition, regardless of the results of the interview, the student is reviewed in depth by a basic science faculty member, a clinical faculty member, and the Director of Admissions. Regardless of the results of this evaluation, the student is brought to a full Medical School Admission Committee meeting. If the student is not accepted by the Committee, his folder is completely reviewed for the last time by the Director of Medical Education along with the Associate Director for Admissions. Every year several alumni children are given acceptances through the recommendations of the Director of Medical Education.

Approximately one out of three alumni children who apply is offered a place in the following fall's entering class. No preference is given for children of physicians who are not Duke alumni, although a surprisingly large number of such individuals are offered places in each entering class. This appears to be due both to the quality of their educational preparation and their familiarity with the demands of the profession.

Comparison of admissions experience between two curricula

The effect of the introduction of the elective curriculum at Duke cannot be separated from other variables which have shaped the experience of the Admissions Committee over the past fifteen years. It may be assumed, however, that the curriculum is among the variables responsible for any significant change in application patterns. Accordingly, comparison has been attempted using three standards: the geographical origin of students, the origin of students by undergraduate college or university, and the final choice of students accepted both at Duke and other representative medical schools.

From 1961 to 1975 the number of applications to Duke per year rose 652 percent, with the largest numerical increases coming from the more populous states, from North Carolina, and from foreign countries. The geographical origins of the students who enroll, with the exception of the special case of North Carolina, are more diverse than the percentage of applicants from each state would indicate (see Table II–7).

Table II–8 describes the origins of recent entering classes by population environment. Although data for comparison with the earlier period are not

Table II–7. Geographical origin of applicants, classes entering during two five-year periods: 1961–65 and 1971–75 (enrollees are noted in parentheses)

State of origin	1961	1962	1963	1964	1965	1971	1972	1973	1974	1975
Alabama	6	9(3)	15	8(1)	7(1)	26	34(2)	22(1)	41	39(3)
Alaska	0	0	1(1)	1	0	0	0	1	1	0
Arizona	2	6	1	3	2	9	18	24(2)	21	31
Arkansas	1	1(1)	2(1)	2	3	4	11	10	8	6(1)
California	57(3)	40(1)	44(1)	52	63(2)	152(4)	262(2)	324(7)	371(3)	492(7)
Colorado	3	2	6	4(2)	6	9(1)	16	27(3)	44(1)	39(1)
Connecticut	17	14(2)	13(2)	38(2)	25	57(1)	83(3)	101(1)	131(2)	119(3)
Delaware	1(1)	1	4(1)	9(1)	3	13	14(1)	7(1)	14	22
Florida	38(7)	43(10)	49(9)	63(9)	72(4)	92(8)	160(5)	151(3)	170(6)	221(5)
Georgia	19(1)	16(2)	24(5)	31(2)	28(4)	71(10)	98(11)	76(3)	82(5)	78(3)
Hawaii	2	0	1(1)	1	1	4	4	9	17	14
Idaho	1	2	3	0	2	3	3	9	7	6
Illinois	13(1)	22(1)	24(2)	33(2)	43(3)	66	84(2)	110(1)	127(2)	137(2)
Indiana	8(2)	8	5	13(2)	10(2)	32(3)	23(1)	35(2)	21(1)	35(1)
Iowa	3	5	4	2	2	15	21	16	12(1)	13
Kansas	2(1)	3	4	9	7(1)	18	23	31(1)	19(2)	32
Kentucky	7(1)	12(2)	13(2)	23	20	21(3)	34(1)	16(1)	37	13(2)
Louisiana	0	3	4	7	3	26(3)	33	32(2)	23	19(1)
Maine	2	3	2	3	3	4	12	15(1)	10	12(1)
Maryland	24(4)	21(5)	72(1)	40(2)	38(1)	68(5)	106(1)	125(4)	132	142(7)
Massachusetts	11	17	25(1)	43(2)	36(2)	94	119(3)	158(3)	175(2)	183(1)
Michigan	9	11	14	14	24	32	50(1)	66	78(3)	82(1)
Minnesota	5(1)	7(1)	1	7	2	19(2)	25(2)	21(1)	33(1)	32(1)
Mississippi	1	3(1)	1	5(1)	3	11(1)	11	15	12	9(1)
Missouri	7	4	4	9(1)	12(1)	29	30(1)	47(1)	42(2)	50
Montana	0	1	2	0	1	2	6	8(1)	6	5
Nebraska	2	1	3	5	2	3	8	5	9	8

	1961	1962	1963	1964	1965	1971	1972	1973	1974	1975
Nevada	0	1	1	2	2	1	0	3	1	2
New Hampshire	1	2	0	1	2	6	7	10	8	12(1)
New Jersey	41(4)	30(2)	63(7)	84(6)	83(3)	118(4)	181(4)	204(7)	237(7)	254(10)
New Mexico	1	3	2	7	1	8	10	19(1)	13(1)	6(1)
New York	103(8)	115(4)	134(12)	222(14)	216(17)	348(10)	550(8)	729(17)	797(10)	892(9)
N. Carolina	71(21)	60(13)	76(15)	77(17)	76(8)	180(26)	250(30)	268(28)	307(36)	316(32)
N. Dakota	0	1	1	1	3	3	1	2	5	5
Ohio	25(5)	33(2)	40(5)	64(4)	47(3)	82(3)	135(5)	143(2)	132(3)	128(2)
Oklahoma	1	4(1)	6(1)	11(1)	7	22(1)	20	24(1)	18	23(1)
Oregon	2	4	3	2	6	9	25	24	30	27
Pennsylvania	42(3)	28(2)	26(1)	72(4)	78(5)	132(2)	179(6)	201(3)	228(4)	206(8)
Rhode Island	2	4	4	10	3	9	12	18	20	22
S. Carolina	19(3)	19(8)	23(3)	14(1)	21(3)	53(10)	63(5)	49(4)	60(10)	44(1)
S. Dakota	0	1	0	0	0	1	2	4	1	3
Tennessee	9(1)	18(5)	21(1)	22(2)	23(6)	32(1)	39(4)	48(2)	61(2)	46
Texas	11	18(2)	19	23(2)	15(3)	48(3)	90(2)	79(2)	64(1)	74
Utah	4	3	5	4	4	18	19	18	20	31
Vermont	0	1	1	2	0	2	6	12	12	10
Virginia	37(8)	41(7)	34(7)	29(1)	49(4)	80(3)	124(9)	120(2)	99(3)	96(4)
Washington	5	3	2	8	7	16	16	38	42(1)	52
W. Virginia	8(1)	22(5)	9(2)	22(1)	11(4)	17	20(4)	19(2)	22	27
Wisconsin	6	3	5	7	8	31	31(1)	33(1)	37	37(2)
Wyoming	0	1	1	1	1	2	3	2	1	1
Other:										
Dist. of Columbia	7	4	8(2)	5	13(2)	16	17	24(2)	18	12
Foreign	14	18(1)	19	16(2)	20(1)	36(1)	63	69(1)	59(5)	77(2)
Total	650	692	799	1131	1113	2150	3151	3621	3935	4242
Class size	(76)	(81)	(81)	(82)	(80)	(105)	(114)	(114)	(115)	(114)

Table II–8. Origin of students enrolled by type of environment, 1973–75*

	Population of 10,000 or less	Population of 10,000–25,000	Population of 25,000–50,000	Population over 50,000
1975–76	27 – 24.11%	18 – 16.07%	13 – 11.61%	54 – 48.21%
	Class of 114 accepted students — 2 foreign students not included			
1974–75	31 – 28.18%	12 – 10.91%	17 – 15.45%	50 – 45.45%
	Class of 115 accepted students — 5 foreign students not included			
1973–74	23 –20.35%	19 – 16.81%	12 –10.62%	59 –52.2
	Class of 114 accepted students — 1 foreign student not included			
Total for 3 years	81 – 24.18%	49 – 14.63%	42 –12.54%	163 – 48.65%

*343 accepted students—8 foreign students not included.

Table II–9. Origin of applicants to Duke by undergraduate college or university: selected years, 1961–75

1961		1965		1971		1975	
College	Number appli- cants	College	Number appli- cants	College	Number appli- cants	College	Number appli- cants
Duke	73	Duke	65	Duke	121	Duke	198
Davidson	24	Harvard	31	Harvard	64	Harvard	117
Univ. of N.C.	20	Univ. of N.C.	28	Univ. of N.C.	56	Yale	105
Cornell	18	Princeton	27	Columbia	51	Univ. of N.C.	104
The Johns Hopkins Univ.	17	Dartmouth	23	Yale	41	Princeton	95
Princeton	17	Rutgers	21	Princeton	38	The Johns Hopkins Univ.	94
Dartmouth	15	Cornell	20	Cornell	33	Stanford	90
Harvard	14	Yale	20	Davidson	33	Cornell	77
Emory	13	Univ. of California	19	Univ. of Pennsylvania	33	UCLA	73
Univ. of California	10	Univ. of Pennsylvania	18	Univ. of California	29	MIT	70

available, the percentage of applicants from urban environments may be declining somewhat and the percentage from rural areas rising.

The data in Table II–9 suggest continuity in the origins of Duke Medical undergraduates, with the major private colleges and universities of the East being the primary sources of applicants. The increased number of applicants per school reflects both the overall rise in the total number of applications and the recruiting trips described above. In the more recent period, southern schools, other than Duke and the University of North Carolina at Chapel Hill, have provided fewer applicants while there has been an increase in the number of applicants from northeastern schools and, more recently, from west coast universities.

The Admissions Committee at Duke, as at other medical schools, must offer more acceptances than there are places in each entering class because some students accepted at Duke will prefer to enroll elsewhere. During the period immediately preceding the introduction of the elective curriculum at Duke, and since that time, there as been no significant change in the number of acceptances offered to fill each class, the only increases coming when the size of the medical school class was enlarged. However, comparison of the final choices made by students accepted both at Duke and at other medical schools does show a significant change when the two periods are compared.

Listed in Table II – 10, for selected years, are the competitive joint acceptances with seven other private medical schools, designated A through G, with whom we traditionally compete for students. The first number in each triplet indicates the number of students having acceptances both from Duke and the designated school. The final number represents the number of students who enrolled at Duke. While percentages vary from year to year, there is a clear and marked increase in the number of jointly accepted students who, since the adoption of the elective curriculum, have decided to accept Duke's acceptance. It seems likely, particularly in view of the data presented in Table II – 1 above, that the elective curriculum is one of the significant factors behind this improved competitive position. Location in a non-urban environment may also be a factor of some significance.

Conclusions

On the basis of the applications experience of the Admissions Committee of the Duke University School of Medicine in the years immediately preceding and following the introduction of the elective curriculum, the following conclusions are offered:

1. There was no significant increase in the number of applications to Duke which could be directly attributed to the introduction of the elective curriculum.

2. In the years since the first students enrolled under the elective curriculum have graduated, the rate of growth of the applicant pool at Duke has increased more rapidly than the national average.

3. The single most valuable source of information about medical schools, according to students entering under both the traditional and elective curricula, is the opinion of students already enrolled at the school.

4. Although change in the relationship between the scores achieved by students enrolled at Duke and the average national score on the Medical College Admissions Test cannot be specifically attributed to the elective curriculum, over the past three years the average score attained by Duke entrants has risen appreciably compared to the national norm.

5. Increased representation of northeastern and western colleges and

Table II–10. Competitive joint acceptances, seven representative medical schools and Duke University School of Medicine, selected years, 1963–74*

Medical school	September entering class							
	1963	1965	1966	1967	1970	1971	1973	1974
A	17–7–2	20–12–3	22–13–2	19–3–8	39–16–1	16–5–1	24–2–5	16–2–2
B	3–1–0	6–4–0	7–4–0	12–6–2	17–3–2	10–4–3	9–3–1	13–5–0
C	5–2–0	8–5–0	18–7–2	12–3–1	25–6–4	9–2–2	16–2–3	19–3–4
D	7–6–1	6–6–0	12–9–2	9–7–0	28–22–1	27–15–2	35–27–4	27–20–4
E	7–5–0	11–2–0	14–7–0	14–8–3	22–8–1	10–7–1	30–12–17	20–7–2
F	7–4–1	5–1–0	11–1–2	10–3–2	11–1–1	4–1–0	10–1–3	8–3–1
G	8–4–0	20–13–0	18–7–2	24–9–6	24–7–2	31–8–9	33–3–9	30–5–7
total	52–29–4	76–43–3	102–48–10	100–39–22	166–70–12	97–42–18	157–50–32	133–45–20

*In each triplet the first figure indicates the total number of students jointly accepted with their medical schools, the second represents the number of students jointly accepted who enrolled at other schools, and the third indicates the number who enrolled at Duke.

universities among applicants to Duke may be related primarily to specific recruiting efforts and to national population patterns.

6. The ability of Duke to attract students holding acceptance to more than one medical school improved significantly in the period following the introduction of elective curriculum.

Basic Sciences

III. Anatomy

J. David Robertson, M.D.

The Department of Anatomy initially was affected more than any other basic science department by the introduction of the elective curriculum in 1966. Where the traditional curriculum had assigned 531 hours in the first year to the teaching of Gross Anatomy, Microscopic Anatomy, and Neuroanatomy, the new proposal provided only 252 hours. There was strong feeling in the Department that students could not be properly prepared for medical careers in less than half the time formerly available, so there was correspondingly strong opposition to the elective curriculum prior to its introduction.

The inauguration of the curriculum coincided with the retirement of Dr. Joseph Markee as Chairman of the Department and the assumption of the chairmanship by Dr. J. David Robertson. Coming to Duke after having devoted most of his career either to Pathology or to full-time morphological research, he had few preconceived notions about how anatomy should be taught to medical students. This absence of prior commitment was an administrative advantage but was a handicap in terms of leadership when it came to generating enthusiasm among faculty accustomed to the traditional structure for teaching within the constraints of reduced contact hours.

Of the 252 hours available, approximately 100 were assigned to Gross Anatomy, an equivalent number to Microscopic Anatomy, and 50 hours to Neuroanatomy, which was integrated with Neurophysiology in a total time allotment of 100 hours. Dr. Talmadge Peele, who had been in charge of the teaching of Neuroanatomy for many years, continued in this responsibility. No severe disruptions or problems occurred in this area, although Dr. Peele constantly felt pressed for time. Microscopic Anatomy had been supervised since 1964 by Dr. Montrose Moses, a cell biologist who, previous to that date, taught in the Research Training Program. Members of the faculty in this area were, like Robertson himself, frequently trained in related areas and new to Duke. This facilitated experimentation with teaching methods and acceptance of criticism offered by either students or staff. By 1971 a stable but flexible structure for the teaching of Microscopic Anatomy emerged, based upon two important points learned during its development.

First, any introduction of basic material in cellular or molecular biology not having a visible, easily understandable and significant connection with the human body structure or system under study was regarded as non-essential and rejected by many, though not all, of the students. Thus, early efforts to have lectures deal with principles of cell biology that underly the structure and function of tissues, and to use the laboratory as an exercise in observing and understanding tissue and cell structure, had to be modified. The first lecture of each topic now presents a selective textbook survey illustrated with microscopic material to be studied later in the laboratory. The second lecture presents the topic in greater detail, elaborating on certain aspects that are considered essential. All lectures are accompanied by complete lecture notes.

Second, the overall curriculum in the first year is highly concentrated, and heavy demands are made on the students' time and attention. In the first semester they must face five separate courses simultaneously, often sitting in lectures or laboratories for all five courses during a nine-hour day. These circumstances determine teaching methods. Students are under heavy pressure and can cope only with the barest essentials; there is little time in which to think or digest, or for free work in the library. Even explicit texts must be abridged, and there is no opportunity for independent study and self-instruction. Under these circumstances the Microscopic Anatomy faculty feels obliged to provide maximum structure. Thus the course is programmed carefully, with objectives made absolutely clear each step of the way. Essential information is supplied in such forms as lectures, lecture notes, selected references to paragraphs in texts, microscopic slide material and audiovisual self-study aids. Laboratories immediately follow related lectures wherever possible.

This system is adequate under the circumstances, and is accepted by the students. Its weaknesses are somewhat offset by advantages provided by the use of teaching laboratories housing eighteen to twenty students. Two instructors have direct contact with such a group of students on the average of four hours per week throughout the course. A new instructor is introduced to the course by sharing a laboratory with a more experienced one. In these sessions instructors exercise considerable autonomy as to how they interact with the students. This usually gives rise to a healthy rapport between instructor and individual students. Each instructor gets to know, and can evaluate, a few students very well.

The major problem developed in the teaching of Gross Anatomy: the staff responsible considered it impossible to cover the subject in 100 hours. After some discussion with various members of the staff and other people in the Medical School, we decided to look at the way in which Gross Anatomy was being taught at Western Reserve University School of Medicine. The people there had had good experience over the years using fetuses for Gross Anatomy dissection rather than adult cadavers. From the information gathered, it seemed a reasonable experiment to try, given the conviction that an adult cadaver could not be dissected properly in 100 hours.

For this experiment, the Central Teaching Laboratories (CTL) were especially equipped with accessory lift-up table tops extending perpendicular to the sit-down height benches. These tops were sufficiently large to hold a tray with a fetus.

The benches were equipped with large magnifying glasses internally illuminated by circular flourescent lights to aid the students in dissecting and identifying the essential structures. In addition, extensive prosections were done in adult cadavers and every part of the body was demonstrated to the students. They were able, in small groups, actually to feel the various structures that had been dissected. Extensive use also was made of audiovisual materials such as models, video tapes, and various films that had been prepared over the years by the previous departmental group under the leadership of Dr. Markee.

The experiment was a complete failure. The students complained endlessly that they could not see what they were supposed to see in the fetuses and that fetal anatomy was different from adult anatomy. Also, four students to a fetus proved to be too many. The faculty complained about the physical facilities. It was impossible to get around in the laboratories to work with the groups of students because of the space required for the accessory tables. The constant complaints from both students and faculty convinced the chairman of the necessity of reorganizing the course.

We decided to try a completely different approach in the following year. We opted to make the course as clinical as possible, since one of the complaints that we had heard from the students was that there was not enough clinical correlation. The entire staff participated in developing a careful outline of the material that was considered to be essential, and this was submitted to all of the clinical chairmen for comments. A strong effort was made to persuade the clinical faculty to participate actively in the teaching of gross anatomy. We decided to abandon the dissection of the fetus and rely entirely on lectures, demonstrations, models, audiovisual material and prosections, because we still believed that it was impossible to dissect an adult cadaver in the time allotted. Good cooperation was obtained from the clinical faculty, and the course seemed to get off to a good start.

We soon realized that this experiment, too, was not working. The main fault was that there was not enough continuity between the lectures. There were too many different lecturers, and practically none of them knew what the previous man had said. The consequence of this was much duplication, and some presentation of inappropriate material. Furthermore, some of the clinical lecturers spent too much time talking about pathological anatomy and too little about the basic principles of anatomy.

We decided then to try a completely different experiment. There was in the department a small nucleus of physical anthropologists led by Dr. John Buettner-Janusch, the Director of the Primate Facility. One of these, Assistant Professor Jack Prost, a primatologist, was well trained in gross anatomy. His research was concerned with that aspect of the body and consequently he was qualified to assume responsibility for the Gross Anatomy course.

Dr. Prost set about the problem in a systematic way. He laid out for himself a very careful and complete plan for dissecting a human body. He then proceded to perform those dissections which he felt were essential, timing each operation. At the end of a total of eighty hours of careful dissection, he had accomplished what he considered to be a sufficiently complete dissection of the cadaver to encompass all of the topics normally covered in the standard course in medical schools. He concluded that the time allocated for gross anatomy was sufficient.

Dr. Prost decided, on this basis, to have the students do a complete dissection of the cadaver in a more or less classical manner. He prepared an outline written especially for the purposes of this dissection. He told the students at the beginning of the Gross Anatomy course precisely what they were expected to do. One crucially important instruction was not to attempt to memorize endless details, such as the origins and insertions of every muscle in the body. For instance, to take an extreme, he told them that he did not expect them to become sufficiently familiar with all the bones of the body so as to be able to reach into a bag and identify the astragulus. He indicated that they should work quickly and efficiently in order to complete the dissections.

Unfortunately, at first this experiment also appeared to have failed. The students seemed quite disturbed and expressed the fear that they were going to be dangerous when they began to deal with patients the next year because of inadequacies in gross anatomy. The chairman spent many hours in the gross lab talking to small groups of students, in order to gain more insight into the situation and to try to reassure them. It soon became apparent that the experiment in fact, had not failed; the source of trouble was not conceptual but rather a problem of personal interactions. Certain of the older staff members were allowing their bias against the new approach to be communicated to the students. They were convinced that memorization of detail was in fact necessary. This affected the students profoundly. In order to deal with the situation, it finally became apparent that some members of the staff had to be relieved of their teaching responsibilities in Gross Anatomy. It was clear that Dr. Prost was addressing the problem in a reasonable manner and that, properly implemented, his method would work. The decision was made, then, to continue along the lines that he had started. The following year, the laboratory manual was revised by Drs. James Shafland and Matthew Cartmill, and this was developed subsequently into a core curriculum textbook for Gross Anatomy. As finally organized, six students work with one cadaver at a dissecting table. There are a few hours spent in lecture-demonstrations and there is a room set aside with adequate supplies of models and audiovisual aids. However, the main emphasis is on the actual dissection of the cadaver by the student himself. This approach has been consistently well received over the years by the students. Reduction of the number of students per cadaver from six to four, when space becomes available, will further improve the results of using this method.

In 1972, the department assumed responsibility for teaching Gross

Anatomy to a group of about fifty physician's associate trainees. In this course Dr. Charles Blake, a neuroendocrinologist, and Dr. Richard Kay, a physical anthropologist, were given responsibility for the Gross Anatomy teaching. They integrated the Allied Health Teaching Program with the medical school teaching in a manner such that the medical students' dissections are examined by the Allied Health students after the medical students complete the dissections. There is much more lecturing and demonstration and use of audiovisual aids in the case of the Allied Health students than in the case of the medical students.

The initiation of the elective curriculum coincided with the appearance of an increasingly vocal generation of activist medical students who demanded explicit relevance of the curriculum to their career goals. During the years just described the curriculum was not merely a scapegoat; it contained a number of genuinely irritating factors, some inherent in its design and some the natural consequence of change and adjustment. On balance, however, the effects of designing a new structure for the teaching of anatomy have been positive. The majority of medical students elect courses in anatomy, and particularly gross anatomy, in the third year. These courses, taught both by the full-time anatomy faculty and joint appointees in clinical departments, are popular with the older members of the faculty because the subject matter can be handled in depth. Joint appointments allow close correlation of studies in anatomy with clinical medicine; for example, an orthopedic surgeon teaches a course on the anatomy of the extremities, and a neurosurgeon gives a course in surgical neuroanatomy. Advanced courses in microscopic anatomy appeal more to graduate students than to medical students.

The reduction of clock hours in required courses has freed members of the anatomy faculty for graduate teaching, research, and undergraduate tutorial teaching. Against these advantages must be weighed the continuing conviction of the faculty that they and the students would find the required courses more satisfying if the time spent in all three categories of anatomy were increased. Final evaluation will be made only as we see what kind of doctors our medical students become.

IV. Biochemistry

Robert L. Hill, PH.D.

Introduction

The major objective of a course in medical biochemistry is to introduce students to fundamental principles important in the study of medicine. This includes a consideration of the structures and functions of the simple, organic compounds of cells. The more complex macromolecules uniquely characteristic of living things, including proteins, nucleic acids, polysaccharides and the complex lipids, are then examined. In addition, special attention is given to the ways chemical processes proceed in biological systems to provide the energy needs of life. In presenting the fundamental principles, it is anticipated both that students will obtain a knowledge of the subject as it exists today and that they will develop a sufficiently sound way of thinking in molecular terms so that they will be prepared to integrate biochemical knowledge into the other basic and clinical sciences studied in subsequent years. Because biochemical information appears to be doubling about every eight years, it is also essential that students be prepared to learn new information as it emerges and to assimilate it intelligently into the knowlege that is required to be an effective physician. To achieve this objective the concepts of biochemistry as presented throughout the course are related, insofar as possible, to questions of clinical importance.

Some practical problems arise on attempting to achieve these objectives in an introductory course, and merit brief comment. First, the question continually asked by students and instructors alike is, What aspects of biochemistry must be well understood in order to be a good physician? No simple answer to the question is possible, but it is clear that in designing a course in medical biochemistry, those aspects of the subject must be considered that are not only immediately useful but also essential if students are to be prepared to learn more biochemistry in the future. In achieving this end, the time devoted to exciting new areas of biochemistry at the "burning edge" of modern research must be limited in order to have sufficient time to present adequately such traditional subjects as nutrition or acid base balance, which are as important in medicine today as they were twenty-five years ago.

Secondly, there is the problem posed by the diversity of undergraduate training of first-year medical students. Some students have sufficient undergraduate training in chemistry and biology to grasp biochemistry without difficulty, whereas others have at best a minimal scientific background to cope intelligently with the course. Other students have had previous course work in biochemistry and it may be difficult to assess whether they should be required to repeat a course in medical school. For the most part, special tutorial assistance has solved some of the difficulties encountered by students with a poor background in science, and a special examination designed by the National Board of Medical Examiners has identified what has proved to be a small number of students with adequate preparation in biochemistry.

Finally, the quality of instruction is a source of major concern. Modern biochemists, as scientists in general, are often so specialized within the field that it is difficult to find a generalist who can bring together effectively the principles of the subject as a whole. In addition, most of the biochemistry faculty are not clinically trained and are reluctant to attempt to discuss medically related questions in their field. For the most part, this has been solved at Duke by insisting that those teaching medical biochemistry become generalists and interact with clinicians in order to cope with the problem of correlating medicine with biochemistry.

These objectives and problems in teaching medical biochemistry have been recognized for many years and were not uniquely associated with the change in the Duke curriculum. Nevertheless, in accommodating to the elective curriculum certain fundamental changes in the design of the course became necessary, as discussed below.

The first-year biochemistry course

Table IV–1 summarizes the kinds of teaching activities in the first year course in medical biochemistry under the traditional and elective curricula and indicates the time allotted to the various course components. Because the structure of the course has changed somewhat from year to year, the table summarizes the design of the course in the first two years (1966–68) and how it has changed over eight years' experience with the elective curriculum.

In the pre-1966 curriculum the biochemistry course was designed along traditional lines. It was given in one semester over a twenty-week period with three hours of lectures, two hours of small group conferences and six hours of laboratory per week. Thus, each student had a total of about 220 contact hours in biochemistry. Between 1961 and 1966 considerable revision was made in the laboratory portion of the course. Clinical-biochemical correlation conferences were built around 6 major laboratory sessions. Each session was given over three consecutive days and students devoted essentially all of their time during these three-day sessions to biochemistry. The experiments were designed to introduce the student to modern biochemical techniques and to provide not only practical laboratory experience in a major area within

Table IV–1. Components in the first year course in medical biochemistry and the time devoted to each component

	Contact hours devoted to each component (percent of effort)			
	Traditional curriculum (prior to 1966)	Elective curriculum		
		(1966–68)	(1969–72)	(1973–75)
Lectures[a]	58 (27%)	50 (31%)	52 (38%)	56 (48%)
Laboratory[b]	120 (55%)	75 (47%)	0	0
Group conferences[c]	40 (18%)	25 (16%)	25 (18%)	29 (25%)
Clinical correlation[d]	0	10 (6%)	15 (11%)	32 (27%)
Seminar[e]	0	0	10	0
Preparation for seminar[f]	0	0	35 (26%)	0
Total hours	218	160	137	117
Length of course	20 weeks	14 weeks	13.5 weeks	13.5 weeks

a. Lectures are presented only once to all students in the class. Approximately three lectures per week were given in the traditional curriculum and four per week are given in the elective curriculum. Until 1966 up to thirty graduate students were enrolled in the course along with seventy-five medical students. In 1967 the course was limited to medical students, although up to six special Ph.D. students from other Basic Medical Science Departments such as Pathology and Physiology have been enrolled.

b. Before each student spent about six hours per week (two half-days) for twenty weeks in the laboratory. In 1967 each student had six major laboratory blocks spaced at intervals throughout the semester. Each block was twelve to fifteen hours in length and was given over three consecutive days.

c. A group of eight to twelve students are assigned one conference instructor and meet with him two to three hours per week throughout the course. The major purpose of this conference is to discuss and review lecture material. At least six hours of this time are devoted to informal, unrecorded examinations. They are intended to be learning examinations for students' self-evaluation.

d. The entire class meets together for biochemical-clinical correlation conferences. The conferences are given by at least one biochemist and one clinician in ten different sessions throughout the course.

e. Each member of a conference group, after consultation with the conference instructor, chooses a special subject in which he is particularly interested and writes a short paper on the subject. Each student then gives an oral presentation of his paper in a special seminar composed of the members of the conference group.

f. All students in the course are given time during the first semester calendar for preparation of a paper in a special area of biochemistry and for oral presentation of the paper in a seminar.

biochemistry but also the opportunity to correlate this experience with clinically relevant problems. For example, protein chemistry was taught in one three-day laboratory session by examining normal and abnormal human hemoglobins in detail and relating the laboratory work and lecture material to the present knowledge of certain hemoglobinopathies and special disorders of the erythrocyte. In other sessions, metabolic experiments employing isotopic tracers and modern metabolic techniques were considered in view of such diseases as gout, diabetes, or cancer.

No major changes in the general objectives in teaching biochemistry were made in adopting the elective curriculum, but the length of the course was shortened from twenty to thirteen weeks, or by about 30 percent. Accordingly, fewer contact hours were available and considerable redesign of the course became necessary. Reduction in direct contact hours was achieved by a modest decrease (about 10 percent) in lecture time and by major reductions in laboratory and conference time, each by 40 percent. Reduction in the laboratory was achieved by giving only four of the six three-day laboratory sessions which had been given theretofore. In view of the apparent success of the clinical-biochemical correlation conferences, which were designed around the laboratory experiments, somewhat more time was formally given to these conferences in order to present material from those sessions which had been eliminated by loss of laboratory time.

After three years of experience with the core year, the faculty of the Department decided reluctantly to drop the laboratory portion of the course. The exact value of the laboratory in a course in any experimental science has been the subject of much debate and a full analysis of the role of laboratory teaching cannot be given here. It was clear, however, that loss of the laboratory would limit not only the scope of the course but also the biochemical education of many students, especially those who intended to carry out independent study and research in the future. Nevertheless, in view of the vast amount of subject matter which is covered in the core year of the new curriculum most students felt they could ill afford much laboratory work. The return in apparently useful information was inherently far less per hour of laboratory time than in an equivalent amount of time in either independent study or the classroom. Certainly, learning in the laboratory is vital to a thorough understanding of an experimental science, but it is also a luxury which cannot easily survive effectively in an accelerated curriculum.

The hours formerly devoted to laboratory work were used between 1969 and 1972 for small group seminars. About halfway through the course each member of a conference group, after consultation with his instructor, chose a special subject of interest and after appropriate library research wrote a short paper on the subject. About thirty-five hours in the first-year schedule were provided for the necessary library work. Each student then presented a twenty- to thirty-minute report based on his research paper before a seminar group composed of students in his conference group and the conference instructor. These seminars were held during the last week of the course.

Although the seminars did not provide the same kind of experience as the laboratory, they served many useful functions. They gave the student the opportunity to consider in depth a special area of biochemistry, which is usually of immediate relevance to clinical medicine. Since the reports often considered areas not covered thoroughly in either the lectures, the conferences, or the text, they helped to expand a student's biochemical knowledge. The seminars also acquainted the student with the biochemical literature and eased the task of using this vast amount of material in the future. Finally, and perhaps most important, they allowed the student to learn, at least in part, something of the experimental method, including its logic, its execution, and its use in collecting new information.

By 1973 other basic science courses also began requiring research papers but provided little or no extra time for their preparation. The faculty in the Department of Biochemistry felt that the seminars generally were a good learning experience, as did most students, especially those with a special interest in the basic sciences or medical research. Nevertheless, many students had insufficient time to devote to preparation of the seminars and the quality of the effort for as many as a third of the class was below the expectations of the faculty. Accordingly, the seminars were dropped from the course. Some of the hours freed as a result of this decision were devoted to additional biochemical-clinical correlation conferences and some reallocated to the genetics course, which had insufficient time in the curriculum.

Table IV–2. Subject matter of the lectures and the biochemical-clinical correlation conferences in medical biochemistry

Subject	Number	Conferences[b]
Protein chemistry	4	1. Sickle cell anemia — hemoglobinopathies
Enzymology	4	2. Hemophilias
Metabolism		3. Iron deficiency anemia
General considerations	2	4. Diabetes
Carbohydrates	8	5. Gout: Lesch-Nyhan syndrome
Lipids	4	6. Glycogen-storage diseases
Energy production	6	7. Antibiotics
Nitrogen	4	8. Metabolic & respiratory acidosis
Proteins & nucleic acids	6	9. Autoimmune diseases
Integration	2	10. Phenylketonuria
Physiological chemistry[c]	11	11. Galactosemia
		12. Malnutrition
		13. Alcoholism
		14. Drug-induced hemolytic anemias
		15. Cancer
		16. Lipid-storage diseases
		17. Acid-base balance
Total	51	

Lectures[a]

a. These are given in the order listed for the most part.
b. Ten to fourteen are given per semester. Representative examples of subjects considered are listed.
c. This includes acid-base balance, hemoglobin, erythrocyte, iron metabolism, plasma proteins, bile, blood clotting, immunochemistry, and related subjects.

Table IV—2 summarizes the subjects covered in the lectures and the clinical correlation conferences in the course as now taught. The scope and the content of the biochemistry course have changed somewhat from the old curriculum. Several subjects that are considered in detail in the present textbook for the course (*Principles of Biochemistry*, A. White, P. Handler, and E. L. Smith, McGraw-Hill, Inc., 5th ed., New York, 1974, 1296 pp.) are not covered in class. These include such subjects as photosynthesis and the biosynthesis of many important cellular constituents such as some of the amino acids, the complex lipids, and the oligosaccharides. Topics such as the chemistry of lipids, proteins, amino acids, nucleic acids, and carbohydrates are not considered in as much detail as under the traditional curriculum. Others—for example, the pathways and regulation of metabolism—receive about as much attention as in the past.

Many subjects are given greater emphasis because of the advances in molecular biology which were first incorporated into the biochemistry curriculum during the 1960's and tended to replace the traditional subject matter of physiological chemistry, such as acid-base balance, the erythrocyte, blood clotting, plasma proteins, and nutrition. Nevertheless, these latter topics remain important, and they are given attention each year both in lectures and in the clinical correlation conferences.

The biochemical-clinical correlation conferences serve a vital function in the course. They are an excellent means of reinforcing fundamental biochemical concepts which are so necessary for an understanding of the molecular basis of disease. In many instances patients are presented, while in others visual aids are sufficient to describe the disease. It should be emphasized that no attempt is made to impart purely clinical concepts, such as diagnosis, management, and treatment. Although these concepts may be touched upon, the conferences are principally a vehicle to teach human biochemistry in a medical setting.

Evaluation of the first-year course

No attempt was made by the faculty in Biochemistry to pretest the content of the first year course, nor were any provisions made to evaluate whether students learned as much biochemistry under the new format as under the old. Most of the faculty in the Department believe that the course content is adequate for a core curriculum. By modifying the course somewhat from year to year in light of self-evaluation and student evaluation of departmental teaching, it should be possible to continue to give a course which meets the needs of medical students.

The only information of an objective nature for evaluation of whether students are learning sufficient biochemistry is provided by the performance of Duke students on the Biochemistry portion of the Part I exam given by the National Board of Medical Examiners. In 1966 and 1967, Duke's rank on the biochemistry exam was twentieth and thirty-fourth. In 1970 and 1971, Duke's rank in Biochemistry was twelfth and fifteenth. Although this performance cannot be taken as a direct reflection of the success or failure of either the new curriculum or the Biochemistry course, it does give the faculty in the Department some reassurance that students do learn a substantial amount of biochemistry compared to a national norm.

Biochemistry electives in the Advanced Science year

Advanced study for third-year students may be obtained through either course work, independent study including laboratory research, or participation in special interdisciplinary programs which are taught at least in part by faculty in the Biochemistry Department.

The courses in biochemistry for third-year students include all of those given in the Graduate School. The Department has had an active Ph.D. training program for over thirty years and since 1960 has had an average of about fifty-five graduate students in residence each year. Because the Department had a strong graduate program when the elective curriculum was implemented, a wide variety of advanced courses was already available for third-year students and no new or special course offerings had to be designed.

Opportunities for independent study and research in biochemistry vary widely and are directly related to the research interests and current research programs of the faculty. All members of the faculty are engaged in active research programs which are supported by funds from external agencies. The types of research now in progress encompass a wide variety of special areas of biochemistry, including protein chemistry, enzymology, lipid chemistry, intermediary metabolism, molecular genetics, X-ray crystallography, neurochemistry, immunochemistry, carbohydrate chemistry, membrane biochemistry, human genetic defects, blood clotting, and biological oxidations. Any third-year student, by special arrangement with individual faculty members, can devote all or part of his third year to independent study in any of these research areas. This may involve library research but experimental work in the laboratory is highly recommended.

Many faculty in the Department are also members of the instructional staff of the interdisciplinary programs designed specially for third-year students. Biochemists are presently involved in the research training program in cell biology, as well as in the study programs in virology, immunology, neurosciences, and growth and development. These programs are described in subsequent chapters.

It is noteworthy that few medical students elect to take advanced biochemistry courses in the third year. Over an eight-year period, an average of twelve to fifteen students per year have elected biochemistry courses in their advanced science year, in addition to the students enrolled in the Medical Scientist Training Program. It is difficult to assess exactly why students do not elect more advanced biochemistry courses but a variety of factors may offer partial explanations. First, biochemistry is apparently, in the minds of some, difficult to relate to career plans. Second, some medical students are reluctant to compete in courses with graduate students, who are far better prepared in chemistry than they. Finally, the Biochemistry Department has been reluctant to design special elective courses for third-year medical students. Although the subject matter appropriate to such courses is currently taught in the graduate program, many medical students are reluctant to devote an entire semester, which is the equivalent of two eight-week elective medical school terms, to a single graduate course. It is of interest that one eight-week course in nutrition was offered by the Department beginning in 1973. In the first year twelve students enrolled, and in the second, twenty-two. Preregistration for 1975 indicates that the course may have still more students, even though a similar course was introduced by the Department of Physiology in 1974.

Staff requirements for teaching biochemistry

New staff were not required to teach biochemistry in the new curriculum. At least fifteen faculty members participate in the first-year course. Between three and four senior faculty give a majority of the lectures and ten or eleven different staff members lead the conference groups. Of particular importance is the participation of clinically trained biochemists in the clinical correlation conferences. This is possible because the Department has had six to eight faculty members with joint appointments in Medicine or Pediatrics who are sound, competent biochemists as well as clinicians. Although these individuals do not give the majority of the conferences, at least one is present at each conference to present a patient, describe the disease under consideration, or direct the discussion.

Comparative evaluation

In changing from the traditional to the elective curriculum there were both losses and gains with respect to the teaching of biochemistry. Prominent among the losses are the sharp reduction in contact hours, the loss of laboratory instruction, and the lack of sufficient time to explain thoroughly how biochemical information is collected, analyzed, and used. Among the gains, it appears that students are learning sufficient biochemistry and judging from National Board performances, may even be learning more biochemistry under the new curriculum. Another positive effect of the new curriculum is the discipline involved in using efficiently the time that is available. Finally, students who wish greater exposure to biochemistry have a much more varied set of opportunities through both the special study programs and independent study.

V. Physiology

Daniel C. Tosteson, M.D.

Introduction

The development of the new curriculum at the Duke University School of Medicine seems to me, in retrospect, more an historical happening than an experiment, at least in the sense that the word experiment is used by a biological investigator. Perhaps this is because my arrival at Duke, in the fall of 1961, coincided exactly with discussions concerning the possibility of elaborating the Research Training Program model, described in an earlier chapter, into combined degree programs in a variety of fields. During my tenure at Washington University I had become convinced that, whatever else the goals of medical education might be, the goal of somehow transmitting to students one set of information which all graduates must grasp and retain was increasingly unrealistic. I was not much interested in mounting a major effort at curriculum revision for the benefit of only a small fraction of students, some of whom already were dropping out of medical school for up to a year to delve more deeply into basic medical science or for several years to complete a Ph.D. However, when other department chairmen (and the fact that the new curriculum was planned initially by chairmen played no small part in its eventual acceptance) responded positively to my conviction that the curriculum should offer opportunities to all students to explore some aspect of medicine in greater depth, I was excited by the possibilities.

I found that my colleagues in the Department of Physiology and Pharmacology also were challenged by the question of how to provide both breadth and depth in medical science education. The physiology curriculum as it existed in 1961 featured laboratory exercises, mainly in mammalian physiology broken down by organ systems, with virtually no elective component. There was no attempt to divide the experience between a component devoted to exposing the students to the language and subject matter of the discipline and a component directed to exploring some one area of the material in depth. The attempt to transfer a large mass of information about most aspects of physiology left no time for the latter process. We resolved to redefine our educational goals. We reduced our committment to breadth of coverage to make opportunity to study some aspect of physiology in depth.

Pretesting

The underlying concept which the department expressed in its curriculum was separation of the exposure component, concerned with language-learning and familiarity with a core set of information, from a tutorial component intended to provide the opportunity to behave like a scholar. Although the latter goal eluded precise definition, it involved extracting from a large body of information that which was useful for present purposes and being able to appraise evidence critically in relation to hypotheses. We made this separation in the belief that one comes to feel the life of science only through the process of learning carefully about a limited subject, and this ideal was impossible in a curriculum devoted exclusively to exposure.

Under the old curriculum some sixteen weeks were assigned to physiology. Beginning in the spring of 1963, we used this time to pre-test material for the new curriculum. The sixteen weeks were divided into a core portion of ten weeks and a tutorial segment of six weeks. The core sequence was based upon the principle that all of the material the students were required to learn would be included either in lectures (numbering approximately forty) or in accompanying lecture outlines. This forced a useful discipline upon the faculty as we sought to define what, of all the material students could learn about physiology, they should learn in their first exposure.

The core portion was divided into six sections, one on general physiology, which described the physico-chemical basis of physiological phenomena, and succeeding units on respiration, circulation, absorption and excretion, endocrinology, and neurophysiology. Laboratory exercises were reduced, and used to highlight or reinforce lecture material. We attempted, in short, to maximize the "take" on a very carefully delimited body of information, and to obtain feedback through conferences and quizzes. A final exam at the end of the ten weeks ended our attempts to assess the breadth of student knowledge.

After the core sequence, each member of the faculty offered a tutorial on some limited theme in physiology during the final six weeks of the course. A list of available faculty and subjects was posted, and student and faculty preferences were matched to create groups of six students each. The growth of the department, from seven in 1961 to ten in 1962 and upward thereafter, was essential to this mode of teaching. The small groups met two or three times weekly to review original papers on the group theme. All members of each group read the papers, each in turn reporting to the group on one paper. The group then discussed the content of the paper, the methods used in research, and the structure of the paper itself. In addition, each student prepared an essay on a limited subject within the theme area. These essays showed a remarkable range of interest and degree of originality, they excited students and faculty alike, and they supported our desire to include a substantial independent study component in the new curriculum.

The period of pretesting, from 1963 to 1965, perhaps was more successful than any other in terms of attracting students to physiology. Under the old curriculum, students were not as heavily committed to other subjects during the time when they were taking the course in physiology. Consequently, they had more time to master the information in the core sequence than in the years following. Also, the novelty of the venture was exciting to both students and faculty.

Beginning in 1966, when the new curriculum was introduced in all departments, the core lecture sequence became, with modification, the physiology component of the first basic science year and the tutorials became the basis for third-year elective physiology offerings. The neurophysiology unit was detached and together with neuroanatomy, taught as part of a three-week block. The remaining five units were taught in approximately the same number of clock hours as during the pretesting period, but the hours were spread out over fourteen weeks. This schedule allowed students a more extended exposure time but, because they now were confronted with core sequences in several departments simultaneously, the overall effect was to increase rather than decrease the learning demands imposed on the students.

The core sequence and the importance of limits

In order to cope with what once again looked like information overload, each student in physiology was assigned to a small group of eight to ten students for weekly review under the guidance of a faculty member and a graduate student. In part with the aid of this device, most students coped effectively with the vast amount of information they encountered in the first year. Not all faculty were enthusiastic about it, however, since they frequently had to deal with students in subjects outside their areas of specialization. The students recognized more readily than some of the faculty that the experience of working together at learning was more important than the level of expertise shown in presenting the material. Only agreement that it was essential for at least one member of the department to know each student well made the review sessions tolerable for these colleagues. Following lectures, conferences by specialists in the area of the lecture topic also helped to reduce this source of anxiety.

Beginning about 1969 an increasing number of students, when asked in these groups to evaluate the core course in physiology, reported that although they found the course well organized and competently presented, they were not excited or challenged by it. In an effort to reinvigorate our medical education effort, we decided to give a new group of faculty the primary responsibility for the course beginning in 1972. Reexamination of the originating concepts accompanied the transfer of responsibility. The new team eased considerably the principle of rigorous definition of the required material, and dropped the lecture outlines in favor of recommended textbook readings.

The problem of how best to define informational goals in a core course is a continuing one. In this case, student response to indefinite limits was decidedly negative. By 1975 primary reponsibility for the course passed once again to a new team. This group restructured the course to include five lectures weekly, and once again defined the core in terms of material in the morning lectures. Students also attended two conferences each week, led by specialists in the areas of the lecture topics, where basic science material was correlated with clinical applications. Faculty time for individual tutorials was made available on demand. An outline, accompanying each lecture, specified behavioral objectives for the students.

A group of approximately twenty faculty and students is working toward the development of sets of 250 – 300 multiple choice questions to define the content of each section of the course. As these sets are perfected, they are fed into a PDP–15 computer for use by the students on an individual basis. Student reponse to the course seems to improve with each successful effort to delimit the required material.

The Advanced Science year

In the earliest discussions among the faculty about the mechanics of the third year there was general agreement on the need for an experience of investigation in depth but lack of consensus on how much free choice students should have in structuring this experience. At one extreme were those who advocated that students should take whatever they wanted from among courses offered by the several departments. At the other were faculty who argued that there be structured themes, or tracks, for students to choose and follow. Within each group there was some disagreement concerning how much of the work load should involve independent research, in or out of the laboratory. Affecting both of these questions was the fact that, although the original curriculum design allowed students to mix basic science and clinical work during the last two years, almost all students concentrated their advanced science in the third year and their advanced clinical electives in the fourth.

At the outset, it was decided that each student would be assigned to the department of his choice. Each department designated a Director of Medical Studies to approve the curriculum of each student and, in theory, to insure that each student would be spending substantial time in independent study. This proved difficult to guarantee, however, particularly in the first few years, both because some faculty did not adhere to the principle and because too many students were too anxious about their futures to accept that amount of independence.

In Physiology we introduced advanced courses, open both to medical students and graduate students, from which individual students could choose. Normally, each member of the department offered one course. In

1968, the first year under this format, one course was offered in clinical physiology and pharmacology, and a majority of third-year students chose this elective.

Faculty dissatisfaction with this enrollment pattern was immediate and widespread, the more so because our experience paralleled that of other departments. It seemed clear that the level of anxiety among students as they came off the wards was too high to allow them to relax enough to take advantage of free elective choice. In particular, demands of residents and interns that students be more broadly knowledgeable during the required clinical year helped to push students toward courses stressing clinical correlations. This only reinforced, however, the tendency of a majority of students to accept as their educational goal the acquisition of information rather than habits and methods of investigation.

In Physiology we had never intended that clinical correlations be confined to one course; accordingly, the clinical physiology and pharmacology course was dropped. The effort of the department now went into developing courses that could be components of what became the study programs. Indeed, department members were very active in the formulation and implementation in these programs. The presence of graduate students in these courses provided sets of peer interactions which upgraded the levels of student performance overall, with students in the combined M.D.–Ph.D. programs bridging between and interpreting the experience of the Ph.D. candidates and medical students.

By 1970, when significant numbers of new curriculum graduates began to serve on the housestaff, peer pressure to redress perceived deficiencies in the information base during the advanced science year lessened and the anxiety of third-year students decreased proportionately. The degree to which students can make free curricular choice thus has increased with the passage of time, confirming to some extent the principle underlying the advanced science year.

Evaluation and projection

On balance, the Duke sequence has worked well. The intellectual challenges of trying to define the information essential to each medical discipline and of constructing multiple-alternative environments where meaningful in-depth investigation can occur are valuable, mind-stretching exercises for faculty and students alike. Tied as it is to the growth of knowledge at one end and to certification and licensing at the other, the issue of making a more explicit informational definition of a medical education will not go away. Duke's attempt to provide an answer that is both definite and dynamic is a helpful contribution.

Effective education, however, like freedom, is a process, not a state. In order for Duke to remain at the forefront of medical education, it is essential for the curriculum to continue to evolve. With regard to the core science year, the issue has been, is, and will remain the definition of contents. This harsh problem is exceedingly difficult for the faculty to address collectively. Perhaps it is just this difficulty in reaching consensus which underlies the academic custom of leaving such judgments about content to individual members of the faculty. However, the core concept requires continuing collective faculty judgments on the information to be assimilated. Another important issue for the core year is the means by which students and faculty can be assured that the designated information has, in fact, been assimilated. In this regard, the translation of core physiology into questions which can be stored in a computer and used by students (an activity now being carried out by Dr. Fellows and his colleagues) has long been attractive to me.

Outstanding problems remain in the advanced science year. The most immediate is that it is still possible for students to float through this year without focusing on anything in depth. Independent study aspects are not stressed sufficiently by all departmental advisors. Although there may be some educational value in a year at a more relaxed pace after the stresses of the two core years, I believe that each student should be required to explore some subject independently and in some depth.

More important, for the long run, is the place of the advanced science year in the overall continuum of medical education. Most students who go into clinical medicine develop, at some point, a real thirst for those aspects of science that bear upon their specialty. The core clinical year, however, is not long enough to permit the development of that kind of taste in all, perhaps even in most, students. At the end of the year, many are still enveloped by the mystique of the clinical setting. Many still are unsure of their career goals. They fear that the advanced science year must be pointed directly to their ultimate specialty to be valuable, and do not appreciate that the process of learning about some subject in depth will be of lasting benefit in their professional maturation no matter what avenue of medicine they enter. The goals described earlier, as they reflect the general value of scholarly scientific activity, seem abstract or remote.

The challenge, then, is to make the benefits of the advanced science year available when they are most desired. In the short run, effort within the advising process to encourage students to mix basic science and clinical experience in the third and fourth years would help students whose career goals are not firm. Similarly, development in the advanced clinical year of study programs similar to those available in the third year would allow students more coherent pathways through the elective years.

More adequate answers can be developed, in the long run, by reconsidering the relationship between medical school and residency training, or alternatively, between medical school and undergraduate education. The first interface is, to my mind, potentially more fruitful. If the M.D. normally were not awarded until after the second year of post-graduate training, and it were required that one year between the third year of medical school and the second year of post-graduate training be devoted to an advanced experience in science, almost all students could elect their science year when they were personally ready for it.

The other alternative, perhaps less attractive, is to require an advanced science year prior to initial clinical experience. Even now many graduates of the better colleges and universities spend time enough in independent study and scientific research before entering medical school that they find the didactic methods of the core science year somewhat confining. Better integration of the last two years of college with the first two of medical school would allow a meaningful elective science year as the culmination of a four-year science continuum. If, after their clinical experience, students wished additional training in basic medical sciences, programs similar to those now offered to clinical fellows could accommodate them.

VI. Genetics

Samson R. Gross, PH.D.

The introduction of a formal course in genetics as part of the elective curriculum at Duke was, in reality, a reorganization and extension of material previously presented fragmentarily in each of the preclinical courses. Failure of the traditional curriculum to provide a systematic introduction to genetics as a discrete discipline was unfortunate because some entering medical students were essentially uneducated in quantitative and molecular biology. Recent upgrading of high school and college science education has produced a better prepared generation of medical students; however, more than 50 percent of the entering freshmen have had little or no formal preparation in genetics, and of the remainder only half recall the basic information they once mastered.

The genetics course as now presented is designed to resolve two related pedagogical problems that arise from the necessity to teach students with widely varied backgrounds but with similar professional objectives. The first involves how best to present genetics to students who have had no previous training without boring that fraction of the class for whom much of an introductory course would be a review. The second is how to present the subject in a manner and sequence that satisfies the common professional objectives of medical students while retaining enough rigor to stimulate further study on the part of those students who have a special interest in the field.

These problems have been resolved, at least partially, by offering a course that draws almost exclusively upon human material to illustrate basic principles and emphasizes those aspects of modern genetics pertinent to medical practice and research. Two methods of presentation are employed: a series of approximately thirty formal lectures covering human general and molecular genetics, and a concurrent series of eight to ten clinical correlation lecture-demonstrations.

The subjects of the lectures include cytogenetics, segregation, assortment, linkage, population genetics, cell genetics, biochemical genetics, the code, nucleic acid structure and synthesis, mutagenesis, and protein synthesis. The clinical correlation series varies somewhat from year to year, but generally includes lecture-demonstrations entitled "Chromosomes in Diagnosis," "Dominant and Recessive Disorders," "Hemoglobinopathies," "Down's Syndrome," "The Genetics of the Clotting Mechanism," "Disorders of

Purine Metabolism," "Xeroderma Pigmentosum," and "Genetic Counseling." Whenever practicable, a patient illustrating the phenotypic consequence of a genetic disease is presented by that member of the staff most familiar with the disorder and the patient. Time also is provided for questioning of the patient (when possible), the physician, and the parents.

Sets of problems illustrating the concepts presented in lectures and demonstrations are distributed periodically to the students for completion during their spare time. Answers are provided only after a reasonable time for attempting the solutions has elapsed. This allows each student to evaluate his or her progress and, if necessary, to seek individual help from the staff. Students are assured that written examinations will be confined to the fundamental operations illustrated by these problems; that is, limited to problem-solving from either statistical or molecular information. We found that, given a carefully delimited body of information to learn and a clear idea of what constitutes adequate performance, students grasp quickly the fundamentals of genetics and become cognizant, at least, of the vast body of genetic information. Examination of students is by written examination at mid- and end-term.

Our overall experience with the presentation of genetics in the framework of the elective curriculum has been gratifying. Genetics can be taught effectively within the allotted time, and even students with a modicum of talent can grasp the essentials. The presentation of patients to the students has proven to be very effective, not only as a teaching aid in genetics per se but also in driving home the social and moral problems raised in patient management and counseling. The mixing of beginning and advanced students, when both groups are motivated by clear clinical correlation of the problems they must solve, is also useful, as those with some prior experience often help those with more meager backgrounds.

VII. Pathology

Thomas D. Kinney, M.D.

William D. Bradford, M.D.

Introduction

Once the decision to develop core courses in the basic sciences was made by the Duke faculty, the Department of Pathology began to experiment with the arrangement and content of the material in its traditional courses. The senior staff was asked to take a fresh and unbiased look at the traditional teaching material and to identify all that was essential to the department's primary responsibility of providing the student with a basic understanding of disease. Decisions were based upon the premise that what is needed for the future practice of medicine is not so much detailed knowledge of specific alterations in each disease process as an understanding of the fundamental biological concepts that are essential to an understanding of all disease processes.

The traditional course had been arranged in two broad categories: General Pathology and Systemic Pathology. General Pathology was taught during the first term of the sophomore year, and Systemic Pathology in the second term. The subject matter is described in Table VII–1. A total of 358 hours was devoted to the course: 92 hours to lectures, 248 hours to various types of laboratory exercises, 10 hours for exams, and 8 hours in orientation. After considerable deliberation, it was decided that the core course could be taught in 205 hours, or 153 hours less than the traditional course. The 43 percent reduction in teaching time was comparable to the reductions required of other basic science courses.

A comparison of the old and new curricula shows that the greatest reduction was in systemic pathology; there was judicious pruning of the traditional subject matter of general pathology as well. It was surprising how much time could be saved in areas such as neoplasia and inflammation by careful planning and rearrangement of subject matter. Ample time was provided for thoughtful and thorough presentation of subject by eliminating repetitious material, such as the slides of rare or unusual tumors that had accumulated in the traditional course over the years.

The important specific diseases and lesions that were formerly taught in systemic pathology were introduced into laboratory sessions to reinforce the concepts presented in lectures. This use of important human diseases to illustrate pathological concepts imparted immediacy and relevance to the laboratory discussions which caught and held the students' interest.

The 1964 decision to delay the elective curriculum until the 1966–67 academic year gave the department two years in which to experiment with the presentation of material in the core form before making a total commitment to the new curriculum. The sophomore course was rearranged to present the proposed core course material during the first 9–10 weeks of the fall term and the remaining portion of the traditional sophomore course during the rest of the year.

To evaluate the new core material, arrangements were made with the National Board of Medical Examiners to give Part I examinations to the students after completion of the entire course. The results of these examinations gave us data upon which to compare the students' knowledge of pathology acquired after the core course alone and after the core course

Table VII–1. Comparison of use of teaching time under two curricula

Traditional curriculum 1964–65		Elective curriculum 1971–72	
I. General pathology 13 wks.	Hours	General pathology 13 wks.	Hours
Introduction & tour	8	Cell injury & reaction to injury	25
Inflammation	20	Circulatory & regulatory mechanisms	16
Disturbances of circulation	16	Inflammation	20
Cellular injury	16	Acute infections	20
Immunopathology	32	Chronic infections	15
Acute infection	18	Patterns of inflammation	26
Chronic infections	18	Neoplasia	27
Viral and rickettsial dis.	16	Immunopathology	20
Neoplasia	64	Metabolic & deficiency disease	25
Genetic & congenital dis.	24	Reading period	7
Metabolic & deficiency dis.	26	Final exam	4
	258		205

II. Systemic pathology   11 wks.

		Summary comparison			
Cardiovascular system	6	Old		New	
Endocrines	9	1964–65	Hours	1971–72	Hours
Respiratory	15	Lectures	92	Lectures	62
GI	9	Laboratory	248	Laboratory	139
GU	6	Exams	10	Exams	4
Reproductive	9	Orientation	8		
Lymphoid & hematopoietic	12	Total	358	Total	205
Bone & joint	9				
CNS	15				
	90				

followed by the remainder of the traditional teaching material. Not unexpec-
tedly, there was a significant drop in class averages when the students were
given the National Board after the core course alone. Not only did the class
average drop below the national average but the number of honors was low in
comparison to the national rate of honors, while the number of failures
greatly exceeded the percent of national failures. However, when another
National Board examination was given at the end of the traditional course
after the students had studied the material given in Systemic Pathology, the
class average was significantly above the national average. Also, the percent
of honors greatly exceeded the percent of national honors, while the percent
of failures was significantly below the national percent of failures.

When the first class under the elective curriculum was examined, using the
National Board Pathology Examination, the same pattern of lower average,
fewer honors and higher fail percentage was encountered at the end of the
core course. Again, when the students took Part I of the National Boards
following the third year—that is, after the second basic science year—the
class average was better than the national average and again Duke honors
were significantly higher and failures significantly lower. This suggests that
the time sequence in which the student is presented with the material in
systemic pathology does not significantly affect test performance as far as
National Boards are concerned (Table VII–2).

Table VII–2. Pathology curricula comparison National Board scores in pathology,
1966–70

Md. year	Exam year	Point in curriculum	Duke mean	National mean	Duke honors (%)	National honors (%)	Duke failures (%)	National failures (%)
1966	1964	Part I	82.3	80.5	25.6	14.7	6.4	13.9
1967	1965	Part I	79.8	79.7	6.6	12.6	15.8	16.8
1968	12/65	After core only	77.3	80.9	2	16.6	23	12.7
	3/66	After core + systemic	83.8	79.6	33	12	3.7	17.6
	6/66	Part I	84.2	80.5	31.7	13.4	2.4	13.3
1969	11/66	After core only	71.3	80.6	1	14.3	4.8	13.3
	3/67	After core + systemic	85.9	80.9	41	16.6	2	12.7
	6/67	Part I	82.1	80.8	17.3	14	6.7	12.6
1970	6/67	After core only	75.3	80.8	2	14.6	30	12.7
	6/69	Part I	83.0	80.1	21	13	5.8	14.5

The role of the pathology faculty

Planning for the pathology portion of the elective curriculum was from the
onset a department effort. The decision to involve all members of the
department was based on the belief that for a curriculum to be successful it
must have the support and understanding of the faculty responsible for

teaching it. Because it seemed that the best way to enlist such support would be to bring the entire staff into the planning process at the earliest opportunity, we started with a series of meetings that involved each member of the department in the structuring of both the core course and the third-year electives. The pathology faculty approached this task enthusiastically and readily accepted study committee assignments both inside and outside the department.

Senior staff members were asked to assume responsibility for portions of the core course that fell within their areas of interest and research. When two or more were especially knowledgeable in a particular area, they were asked to form a subcommittee to develop a teaching plan for later review by the entire staff. As a result, we were able to incorporate a variety of teaching approaches into the core course. The student's basic needs in a core course constituted the criteria for selection of topics and the assignment of time to each. Senior staff members whose research or specialty service interests did not coincide with these needs as the entire group saw them were assigned little or no responsibility for teaching in the core course.

Each senior staff member with the rank of Assistant Professor or higher was asked to develop a plan for an elective course. If the suggested elective was accepted, after review by the senior staff as to content and appropriateness, the responsible faculty member was asked to prepare appropriate material such as the syllabus, slide sets, laboratory outline, etc. This freedom to choose both a subject and the way it should be taught was appreciated by the faculty. The professor responsible for a new course invariably approached his teaching assignment with dedication and enthusiasm; it became a matter of personal pride for the teacher to make his course a worthwhile learning experience.

Curriculum planning was shaped by the recognition that the Department of Pathology has two roles to fill. First, it must teach the basic science component that deals with basic mechanisms and pathogenesis of disease. Second, it must cover the large body of knowledge, much of it empirical, that the student must have to approach the diagnosis and treatment of disease in an intelligent manner. This includes the vocabulary of disease. A very practical series of decisions had to be made regarding the allocation of material between the basic core course to be taught in the first year and the elective courses to be taught in the third year. Among the structural questions considered were the amount of repetition of material in the core course and the electives, redundancy among the electives, and the academic level at which material would be presented in an elective when the student returned to the department in the third year with the additional knowledge of pathology gained during second-year clinical experiences.

In our efforts to develop the basic science component of the core course, the staff was mindful of the fact that the basic science courses at Duke, and indeed in most medical schools, overlapped departmental lines. This is because the principles of molecular, cellular and systemic biology are not unique to one discipline but constitute a unifying bridge between all of the scientific disciplines and clinical specialties. In short, while the patterns of disease may be diverse, the underlying biological processes have much in common. Therefore, in planning a curriculum, it is necessary to recognize that too often material is presented in a disjointed, fragmented manner by two or more departments, neither of which has made the effort to find out what the other is teaching. Usually we reached agreement to assign subject matter being duplicated to one department or the other, or to correlate teaching schedules for more organized presentation of material when two departments were found to have somewhat different approaches in a particular area. In either event, eliminating repetitious material saved considerable course time.

The choice of class material relating to clinical practice was a particular critical and difficult instance of this sort. Naturally, the pathology faculty hoped that students would return from their sophomore clinical experiences to enroll in elective courses with a new perspective and with renewed interest. Ideally, a student interested in a career in pediatrics would elect a course in pediatric pathology and one desiring to become an internist would select electives in renal, pulmonary and cardiac pathology and so on. But, since there was no certainty that this would take place, it was necessary to be certain that the core course contained all material considered absolutely necessary for the practice of medicine. Members of the clinical faculty responsible for the teaching of clinical diagnosis and the clinical clerkships were consulted to determine the basic information the students would need to solve the patients' problems they were likely to encounter. On the whole this information was very helpful, although the responses occasionally were anecdotal or too much colored by the experience of an individual clinician. Even with useful guidance, however, many decisions regarding the choice of material to be included necessarily were arbitrary.

When making curriculum changes a teacher's first obligation to his students is to make certain that the new course is at least as good as the one it is replacing, and that it will be taught effectively. Unfortunately, it is very difficult to measure how successful a course is in terms of new knowledge imparted to a student. Even more difficult is the task of determining whether or not the course has led a student to an understanding or appreciation of the basic concepts of a subject so that it will stimulate that student to keep abreast with it after he has completed his course work.

The introductory (core) course

In our new curriculum the student comes in contact with pathology in the second term of the first year. Most of the senior staff members participate in the teaching of this core course, which lasts thirteen weeks. The pathology core course is required for all medical students and introduces the principles of pathology. Emphasis is placed on etiology and pathogenesis of disease and the experimental approach to an understanding of disease. Lectures develop broad concepts of disease processes while laboratory conferences amplify the basic principles taught in the lectures and stress examination of gross and microscopic material with clinical pathological correlation. Each laboratory section of twenty students is supervised by two staff pathologists and a resident to increase personal contact and interchange. In sequence, the core course emphasizes six major areas of general pathology:

1. Cell injury and inflammation   3 weeks
2. Acute and chronic infection   2 weeks
3. Circulatory disease   1 week
4. Metabolic and deficiency disease   2 weeks
5. Immunopathology   2 weeks
6. Neoplasia   3 weeks

During the core course, students are required to take part in postmortem studies, and problems presented by recent autopsies are discussed in small groups in clinical pathological conferences where each student is given a responsible role. We believe that an understanding of the complete biological spectrum is of great value in understanding disease; therefore, the staff devotes considerable effort beyond the material traditionally taught under the heading of general pathology, to principles of cell biology and its relationship to cellular pathology.

Electives in pathology

The elective courses in the third and fourth years at Duke are the raison d'etre for the new curriculum. Electives provide each student with the opportunity to become acquainted with a variety of disciplines related to his career choice. Once a choice is made, the elective system allows study in considerable depth in an area of particular appeal or survey study in several disciplines important to a chosen career.

The students readily accepted the elective curriculum in pathology. Repeated polls of the student body failed to reveal dissatisfaction with the elective system per se, although the students were quite vocal when a particular course did not measure up to expectations. As a matter of fact, pathology electives attracted more students than those of any other basic science. In the years 1968–73, enrollment for pathology elective courses was 1,383, or 34 percent of the total enrollment for electives in the six basic sciences. When the electives were calculated in terms of academic weights or credits based on hours of instruction in lectures, laboratories, seminars, etc., pathology totalled 4,312, or 37 percent of all the academic hours taught in the basic sciences during the study period (Table VII–3). The Pathology Department offered more electives that were chosen by more students than any other single basic science department. The Pathology Department also spent more time and effort on teaching than any other basic science department.

Table VII-3. Pathology electives in relation to other basic science electives

	1968 E/W	1969 E/W	1970 E/W	1971 E/W	1972 E/W	1973 E/W	1968–1973 E/W	Average E/W
Pathology electives	288/972	261/808	233/674	130/385	179/579	292/894	1383/4312	230/719
All basic science electives	715/2167	711/2029	635/1732	468/1197	569/1676	849/2431	3947/11232	658/187
Pathology electives as percent all basic science electives	40/45	37/40	37/39	28/32	31/29	34/37		34/37

E = Enrollment. Number of students taking one or more courses in a given discipline or disciplines.

W = Academic weights taken in a given discipline or disciplines by enrolled students. Weights relate to course hours of instruction; i.e., 1 hr./wk. = ½ wgt or 8 hr./wk. = 4 wgts.

Table VII–4. Pathology electives offered each year by term

All terms			
tutorial—autopsy—surgical			
Term 1	Term 2	Term 3	Term 4
Pathologic basis of clinical medicine	Biochemical	Oncology	Surgical
Ophthalmic	Renal	Environmental disease	Electron microscopy
Cytolopathology	Pulmonary	Core course	Hepatic disease
Cardiovascular neuropathology	Pediatric Exp Cardiovascular		Orthopedic Immunopathology

Terms 1 & 2	Terms 3 & 4
Subcellular and Molecular Histochemistry Pathology of Virus Infection	Hematopathology

Teachers of pathology are always aware that in teaching students they must present both the clinical and basic science components of pathology. The student must be taught those concepts that will provide a basis for understanding fundamental disease processes and at the same time must learn the manner in which functional and structural alterations of cells and tissues are reflected by the clinical manifestations of disease. This dual responsibility demanded two types of electives—one oriented to the basic component and the other to the clinical component. For example, some courses were devoted to the subcellular and molecular aspects of pathology and others were oriented to the clinical practice of medicine in such areas as cardiovascular or renal pathology (Table VII–4).

There is considerable variation in the course content and level of student participation presupposed by pathology electives. Some require the student to present three half-days per week while others require only one half-day. The larger courses are usually taught by several members of the department while the smaller courses are taught by only one or two. Sometimes a course director invites other basic scientists and clinicians to cooperate with him in organizing an interdisciplinary course in some particular field. While each course varies in format and approach, all create opportunities for clinical pathological correlation whenever possible.

Major importance is assigned to three full-time elective courses in pathology that are available in all terms; autopsy pathology, surgical pathology, and a tutorial in pathology. Autopsy and surgical pathology are full-time clerkship electives in which the student assumes direct but supervised responsibility for active case material. The pathology tutorial gives the student an opportunity to work in a one-to-one relationship with a member of the senior faculty. In preparation, the student and instructor make careful plans for a tutorial period that may involve independent research at the bench, collaboration in an ongoing investigation, or library research. By making possible a close relationship with a senior pathologist the tutorial experience brings the student into the mainstream of the department's activities, including research seminars and contact with graduate students in pathology. During the tutorial, a medical student vicariously experiences a career in pathology by "trying it on for size." In practice, the majority of students who elect tutorials in pathology spend full time in our department for one or more terms.

The electives that are most heavily subscribed by the students are those that are most directly applicable to the practice of medicine (Table VII–5). This is not surprising, since most students preparing for the practice of medicine seek a relatively direct road to their goal. Students at Duke are urged, in fact, to make at least a tentative career choice after the second year and to use their electives to prepare themselves for it. As a result, the more popular electives in all departments are usually those that relate most directly to the diagnosis and treatment of disease. In pathology, these are the Pathological Basis of Disease, Cardiovascular Pathology, and Renal Pathology, areas which are essential for the practice of any medical specialty. Electives such as neuropathology, and orthopedic and ophthalmic pathology are chosen by students who are headed for these specialties. Such electives as subcellular and molecular pathology usually are taken by students who have decided definitely upon careers in pathology and by graduate students in pathology and other basic sciences.

Graduate degree programs in pathology

The introduction of the elective system was a great aid to the department in developing programs for graduate degrees in pathology. The Ph.D. program was designed to provide the opportunity for careful study in depth of biology and cellular pathology. In contrast to the resident type of training, the

Table VII–5. Pathology electives enrollment (1968–73)—all students

Course	1968	1969	1970	1971	1972	1973	Total students
Cardiovascular	42	39	29	14	26	43	193
Pathologic basis of clinical medicine	45	27	20	12	35	42	181
Renal	40	29	17	13	11	33	143
Tutorial	9	15	39	24	21	27	135
Pediatric	29	25	26	7	19	23	129
Pulmonary	8	17	25	7	15	33	105
Surgical	25	10	12	10	17	15	89
Autopsy	13	14	5	4	10	13	60

emphasis in the graduate program is not on diagnostic pathology but on the science of pathology. The goal of the Ph.D. program is to produce medical scientists who have a special interest in and knowledge of all disease processes and who are particularly well prepared to do significant disease-oriented research using the most modern methods. Upon completion of their training, they can expect to find many career opportunities as teachers and investigators in academic departments of pathology.

The Ph.D. degree was not offered by the Department of Pathology prior to the advent of the elective curriculum. The new system made it possible to offer a program of great flexibility that would be especially attractive to students interested in experimental pathology, and a research training grant made it possible for the department to support qualified students. During the first five years of the program the candidates were required to have an M.D., a D.V.M., or the equivalent to be accepted. Later students with B.A. or B.S. degrees were occasionally admitted, provided that they had excellent backgrounds in biological science.

In organization the program was quite similar to those offered by other basic science departments in the medical school. Students were encouraged to tailor their electives to meet their needs, particularly in relation to their anticipated areas of research. Initially, however, they were required to devote the greater part of their efforts to formal course work. The goal was to make sure that the candidate attained a thorough understanding of structural changes, their biochemical and physiological relations, and the ultrastructural basis of these processes. After approximately a year and one-half of formal coursework, each student undertook to plan and carry out a research project in an area of special interest. He was allowed to choose his own advisor for the project from the senior faculty of the Pathology Department who were also members of the graduate school faculty. The student was required to meet all the other usual requirements for the Ph.D. degree.

The number of students electing to study for the Ph.D. degree in Pathology was gratifying. The program was opened in the academic year 1966–67 and in 1971 graduated its first students. Since 1971, twenty students have been awarded Ph.D. degrees and there are currently eight students in the program. It is interesting to note that six graduates entered the program with a baccalaureate degree alone, and another six graduates entered after receiving the M.D. degree. Eight graduates entered the training program through the M.D.–Ph.D. program which enabled them to earn both M.D. and Ph.D. degrees at the same time.

In 1972, we decided to offer a Master of Science degree in pathology in the belief that such a program would be of particular value to medical students who wished to take a "year out" while in medical school. It also would enable individuals with baccalaureate degrees to qualify for teaching in the allied health field or give highly motivated technical workers an opportunity to improve their background and skills in a particular area of pathology.

Great care has been exercised in selecting the candidates for this degree to make certain that they are highly motivated and are likely to profit from the program. So far, there have been four graduates, all of whom have expressed satisfaction with the program. However, the faculty feels it is too early to make a judgment regarding the program's ultimate value.

The arrangement and content of Introduction to Pathology, the core course, has been of considerable interest and help to a small number of graduate students from other departments in the university. From 1968 to 1974, nineteen graduate students completed it successfully. Eleven of them have been M.S. or Ph.D. candidates in Pathology; the remaining eight were graduate students in Anatomy and Physiology.

Some started the course at a disadvantage because they had not had the opportunity to take the prerequisite courses in anatomy and histology that normally are required. This difficulty has been overcome by providing such students with study sets of histologic slides of normal tissues and by asking their laboratory instructors to make special efforts to provide them with a working knowledge of histology. The faculty of the department has been glad to see such students interested in pathology because it will give them a broader understanding of disease. As they in turn become faculty members, their better understanding of the science of pathology will enable them to relate to the faculty of pathology departments in medical schools.

The number of graduate students from other departments throughout the university who elected courses in pathology was a gratifying dividend of the new curriculum. It is the opinion of many thoughtful scholars of pathology that the value of some knowledge of pathology has not been recognized by many biomedical scientists. It seems odd that the importance of the relationship of biology to its abnormal counterpart, cellular pathology, has not been appreciated by these scientists, particularly when so much of their time and energy is devoted to disease-related research.

Internship in pathology

One possible gauge of the effectiveness of teaching pathology in the final undergraduate medical years is the number of students attracted to careers in pathology. Consequently, the number of Duke graduates taking internships in pathology after the adoption of the elective curriculum (1970–74) was compared to the number of Duke graduates entering postgraduate pathology training between 1960 and 1964. At that time there was no formal exposure to pathology after the second year other than the Clinical Pathological Conference. From 1970 to 1974, students who interned in pathology numbered twenty-nine, compared to six during the period 1960–64. Under the traditional curriculum, an average of 1.5 percent of each Duke graduating class entered pathology; under the elective structure the comparable figures is 6.8 percent.

In an attempt to determine the preferences of the students who became pathology interns, the course selections made by students in pathology were compared with those of students choosing other careers. Both groups picked electives that were heavily clinically oriented. Students interning in pathology more often elected autopsy pathology, tutorial in pathology, and surgical pathology. The remainder of the student body found the broad courses in systemic pathology and cardiovascular pathology more to their liking. It was somewhat of a surprise to find out that only seven of the twenty-nine students who eventually became interns had elected basic science courses in pathology in the graduate school. This figure became even more striking since five of these seven students were studying for the Ph.D. in pathology and these graduate courses were required.

Of the graduates selecting an internship in pathology fifteen (52 percent) had participated in a tutorial experience as medical students. Many tutorial projects have merited formal presentation at national meetings as significant contributions in experimental pathology. From 1970–74, members of the Department of Pathology read forty-six papers before the annual meetings of the American Association of Pathologists and Bacteriologists. Students were authors or coauthors on twenty-one (46 percent) of them. Nine papers were coauthored by M.D. candidates, nine by M.D.–Ph.D. candidates, and three by students studying for the Ph.D. or B.S. degree alone.

Discussion

The present study indicates that well-organized and well-presented elective courses in pathology are attractive to medical students. The deciding factor for many students in choosing a basic science elective appears to be its perceived relevance to the practice of medicine. This is supported by the finding that students elect more courses in pathology than in any other basic science and that the most heavily subscribed electives in pathology were those that were clearly clinically oriented, i.e., cardiovascular or renal pathology. A significant fact which has emerged from our study is that five times the number of students who have studied under the elective system have elected internships in pathology than was the case under the non-elective system. Also, 6.8 percent of Duke graduates enter pathology, a sharp contrast to 3 percent, the national average of all medical school graduates. This, needless to say, has been very satisfying to the members of our staff responsible for our teaching program.

The reasons given for a career choice are highly personal and are often complex and difficult to evaluate. In one study, a group of 400 pathologists were queried as to considerations which led them to select pathology as a career. The most important was "enjoyment of the challenge of pathology problems." Close behind this was the "influence of pathologists" who were encountered either as teachers or as research mentors. The influence that a teacher has on any career choice is a recurring theme that runs through almost all studies of reasons for a career selection.

If a student is in the Pathology Department attending lectures and seminars or working in the laboratories he will be forced to think about pathology. It will be a very dull student indeed who will not arrive at some decisions as to whether he likes or dislikes it. Studies have shown that the majority of pathologists decide upon or at least give serious consideration to pathology as a career before leaving medical school. The environment in which the student will become acquainted with and judge pathology is largely controlled and determined by the teachers of pathology. Therefore, the teacher will be largely responsible for the student's attitudes toward pathology for the remainder of the student's career in medicine; friend or foe, the teacher will decide.

The elective system as developed at Duke follows the university concept of offering the introductory general course with a wide selection of courses for the study of specific areas of the field in depth. Since the electives are taught by members of the department who have a special competence in the subject matter and since presumably the student who selects the elective has a special interest in the subject matter, it is not surprising to find that the students develop considerable rapport with their teachers. Here, then, we have developed the situation in which "enjoyment of the challenge of pathology problems" and "influence of pathologists" are both present. Certainly the teachers who had freedom to develop the electives in the manner that was most suitable to their type of teaching were pleased and have always indicated satisfaction with their teaching assignments. Some of their enthusiasm for their subjects is in turn transmitted to their pupils.

We are not suggesting that the elective system is the only reason so many students selected careers in pathology. We are saying that bringing the student back to the pathology department after some clinical experience provides pathologists with an opportunity to present pathology in a new perspective. Whether the student spends his time in a clerkship in surgical pathology or in autopsy pathology, taking electives per se is probably less important than developing an appreciation of the practice of pathology and its role in patient care. The major advantage of the elective system is that it permits many more students to participate than can be handled by clerkships. In our department, at least, it is not possible to accommodate more than two or three students on the surgical pathology or autopsy services at a time because to take more would put the students in competition with the resident staff for the fresh pathological material. On the other hand, it is not uncommon for twenty to thirty students to sign up for the more popular general electives and five to ten for the more specialized electives. This means that most of the students in any single class are in our department of pathology during the school year. This may be why the elective system, or any arrangement that brings students into contact with pathologists during the last two years when they are making career choices, seems to be so influential in recruiting for careers in pathology. The fortuitous combination of a good teacher presenting exciting and relevant material during that critical period may be the factor that tips the balance toward pathology. This the elective system seems to provide.

Reference

1. Thomas D. Kinney et al., *Survey of American Pathologists*. Baltimore: The Williams and Wilkins Company, 1966, *passim*.

VIII. Microbiology and Immunology

Wolfgang K. Joklik, D. PHIL.

Many of the problems with which a general practitioner has to deal concern microbial infections. These range from bacterial infections, where the problem is nowadays principally one of selecting the right antibiotic, to viral infections, the treatment of which is still largely confined to providing relief, and to mycotic and parasitic infections, which require careful diagnosis, shrewd management and thorough follow-up. Straightforward infections generally present few problems. Chronic infections, in which microorganisms are localized in inaccessible locations, or viral infections which may remain latent for long periods of time and provide no antigenic stimulus, thus depriving the body of its chief natural defense, can be difficult to diagnose and frequently require great skill for successful treatment. In order to prepare the medical practitioner adequately for this challenge it is necessary that he acquire, on the one hand, knowledge concerning the fundamental nature, properties and behavior of microorganisms and of the basic principles of chemotherapy and immunology, and on the other, that he develop an understanding of the interaction of pathogenic microorganisms with the human organism and of the implications of the normal and abnormal functioning of the immune mechanism at both the humoral and cellular level.

At Duke the responsibility to define, subdivide, assign and control the material to be taught rests with the individual department; indeed, the tradition of departmental autonomy represents one of the most significant elements of continuity in the transition from the traditional to the elective curriculum. Basic and clinical aspects of both microbiology and immunology have always been taught by a single department at Duke. Consideration of microorganisms and immune phenomena per se and their treatment in relation to human disease have never been divorced, as is the case in medical schools where one is taught by the Microbiology Department, the other by a Division of Infectious Diseases in a clinical department. In fact, the staff of the Department of Microbiology and Immunology at Duke has always encompassed faculty members who complement each other with respect to the basic and clinical approaches of their discipline, or who actually bridge them, and who can therefore teach one integrated course encompassing all aspects of both microbiology and immunology.

Under the traditional curriculum, prior to 1967, the Microbiology and Immunology course for medical students was given in the fall of the second year, from September to December. Its objective was to familiarize medical students with the nature and properties of pathogenic microorganisms, the diseases which they cause, and how to treat these. In addition, the basic principles of bacterial physiology, virology and immunology were considered. Since fourth-year electives were rarely taken under the old curriculum, the second-year exposure to microbiology and immunology attempted not only to lay a foundation for further growth in these disciplines, but also to provide students with many of the practical and applied aspects of the management of infectious disease and immunological disorders which medical practitioners would require at the outset of their career. This was accomplished through a course lasting fifteen weeks and comprising seventy-four lectures and ninety hours of laboratory work which comprised essentially diagnostic bacteriology, mycology and parasitology, together with some exposure to basic immunological techniques. The course was highly successful as judged by students' performance in Part I of the National Board Examinations, which were taken at the end of the second year. Students regularly obtained higher mean scores for microbiology than for any of the other basic science subjects, and the failure rates in this subject, rarely over 5 percent, were the lowest.

When the elective curriculum was instituted, the Microbiology and Immunology course was moved from the first semester of the second year to the second semester of the first year, and was restructured to conform to the concept of a core curriculum. It was decided that for their first exposure to microbiology and immunology students should be provided only with the basic principles on which further learning could be based; this further learning was to be provided in the third year. In addition, although interdepartmental teaching was not introduced, all basic science subjects taught in the new basic science core year were carefully integrated. For example, care was taken not to repeat in the Microbiology and Immunology course biochemical and genetic principles already covered in the first semester, and its immunology section was coordinated with the immunopathology section of the Pathology course. As a result, it proved possible to shorten the course by 20 percent without sacrificing essentials.

The emphasis of the core course in Microbiology and Immunology differed substantially from that of the old course. In particular, greater emphasis now was placed on basic principles rather than on practical applications. The emphasis in the basic bacterial physiology section was changed. Discussion of the biochemistry of bacterial fermentations was covered largely in the Biochemistry course in the first semester. The core course in Microbiology and Immunology provided the background for an understanding of the mode of action of antibiotics and chemotherapeutic agents and an examination of those differences in the molecular biology of bacterial and mammalian cells which might prove exploitable in the future. The basic virology section was expanded in order to prepare students for a rational approach to antiviral chemotherapy and for the possible involvement of viruses in the causation of cancer and slow chronic degenerative diseases. At the same time the number of immunology lectures was reduced, which became possible because of their integration with the immunopathology lectures. The number of parasitology lectures was also reduced. Table VIII–1 describes the utilization of time now available for the basic course. Table VIII–2 compares the use of lecture time under the two curricula.

Table VIII–1. Microbiology and immunology utilization of available time by activity

Activity		Hours
Lectures		67
Laboratory exercises		
(a) Diagnostic bacteriology	27	
(b) Immunology	2	
(c) Virology	8	
(d) Mycology	8	
(e) Parasitology	12	57
Clinical presentations		13
Films		5
Conferences		4
Quizzes		6
Total		152

Table VIII–2. Microbiology and immunology: lecture time, by topic, in two curricula

Topic	Pre-1966 curriculum (course offered in fall of second year)	Post-1966 curriculum (course offered in spring of first year)
Clinical bacteriology	18	16
Bacterial physiology	12	12
Clinical virology	9	7
Basic virology	4	10
Immunology	13	8
Mycology	7	6
Parasitology	11	8
Total	74 hours	67 hours

A total of eighty-three hours is available in addition to lecture time, as shown in Table VIII–1. Under the pre-1966 curriculum the largest portion of this time was devoted to laboratory exercises. Under the post-1966 curriculum laboratories are no longer assigned on the assumption that physicians will have to do their own testing procedures; rather, they are designed to amplify or make concrete the material developed in lectures and to stimulate the imagination of the student. Labs have been retained, for example, in diagnostic bacteriology, mycology, and parasitology, but have been dropped from the immunology section of the course and may soon also be dropped from the virology segment. Overall, the laboratory exercises have been reduced by almost 50 percent. The time gained is now devoted largely to clinical presentations which are popular with the students, provide an excellent framework for participation and discussion, and serve the general purpose of integrating the curriculum.

In designing the core course the faculty have been aided considerably by their responsibility for rewriting and revising, every four years, Zinsser's *Microbiology*. This responsibility, which has overlapped the transition from one curriculum to another, has helped us to clarify our ideas about how best to put across the basic concepts of microbiology and immunology and in deciding what concepts are truly important for core consideration. It has also kept in view the similarities in our objectives under the two curriculum structures, which otherwise might have seemed less similar because of changes in teaching methods.

As can be seen from the foregoing, the new course is not core in nature simply because it represents a condensation of the old course. It attempts to present the core of modern microbiology and immunology so as to give the student what he needs to know in order to understand the advances likely to occur in this field over the next twenty or thirty years, or during the productive phase of his medical career. It now presents a much wider view of the subject, particularly in its increased emphasis on basic and fundamental concepts and on the principles rather than the minutiae of patient-oriented microbiological and immunological practice. It encompasses a large amount of material, but the students respond to it extremely well; they consistently rate the course highly. They reveal a remarkable grasp of the material in the three two-hour examinations administered by the Department, which determine whether or not a student is promoted to the second year. These internal examinations better serve the purpose of the Department under the new format than the old requirement that students take and pass Part I of the National Board Examinations.

Under the elective curriculum the first-year core course is only the first part of students' exposure to the basic medical sciences. After the second or core clinical year, students devote their third year to detailed and advanced study in some basic medical science area of their choosing. There are numerous forms which this study can take. First, students may choose a preceptor among the faculty and work with him on his research projects. This research experience may be supplemented by elective courses related to the research topic. Second, students may enroll in one of about ten programs of either one or two semester's duration. These involve research in the laboratory of a faculty member supplemented by a course of didactic lectures tailored specifically for each program and by a series of weekly seminars in which recent research advances are discussed both for their theoretical and practical implications. Third, students may choose to enroll in several of the courses which the basic science departments offer specifically for the third year, and this didactic experience may be supplemented either by library research or by research work in the laboratory of a faculty member. All combinations of these three basic types of experience are possible; in fact, the third year basic science curriculum at Duke University Medical School now has great flexibility in that any student may supplement his first-year basic science base in any area and in any manner he desires. To date, no two students have chosen exactly the same experience in the third year.

What is true of students generally is true of students interested in working within the Department of Microbiology and Immunology. First, the Department offers two integrated programs, each of one semester duration, one in virology, the other in immunology. Each program involves research in the laboratory of a faculty member with an appointment in the Department, a didactic lecture course on advanced topics and a weekly seminar. Students who participate in these programs in the first semester frequently continue working on the project during the second semester, on a preceptorial basis. Second, the Department offers five courses covering the major areas of microbiology and immunology: Basic Medical Virology, Medical Immunology, Immunohematology, Pathophysiology of Infectious Diseases and Medical Mycology. Third, in addition to offering research experience on a preceptional basis, the Department offers training in practical and laboratory techniques of certain areas of microbiology and immunology in the form of structured courses. These areas are immunohematology, diagnostic virology, diagnostic mycology and diagnostic bacteriology. Finally, all graduate courses offered by the Department are available to third-year medical students and a minority avail themselves of this opportunity.

Among medical students the most popular courses offered by the department are Pathophysiology of Infectious Diseases, which enrolls over 50 percent of the total class in any given year, and Medical Immunology, which enrolls 25 to 30 percent. In general, the attempt to design courses for both medical and graduate students has not been successful. Most medical students want microbiologic concepts explained in terms of situations they will encounter in clinical practice, while graduate students are much less concerned with applications. In any given academic year the two groups will be separate in 75 to 90 percent of their courses. The major exception is the core course for first-year medical students, which is required also of graduate students. The general orientation to the field which it provides serves graduate students as a common experience from which they fan out in pursuit of their individual interests.

Currently there are twelve students in the department participating in the Medical Scientist Training Program. During the first year of their Ph.D.

research experience, which starts in April of their second year, these students fulfill the requirements for the preliminary examination mandatory for all graduate students in the Department. Those requirements comprise courses in bacterial physiology, molecular biology, genetics, virology, immunology, and generally also physical biochemistry. These courses usually consist of lectures and seminars, but may also take the form of weekly meetings with faculty members on a tutorial basis and the composition of weekly literature review papers. Once the preliminary examination has been passed, students move into the laboratories of faculty members for a two- to three-year research experience. Often this experience starts even before the preliminary examination, for it is considered desirable that students should engage in laboratory research as soon as possible.

In summary, the transition from the traditional curriculum to the elective has not been an abrupt one for the Department of Microbiology and Immunology. The authority of the Department in the determination of course content and methodologies, the collateral aid in assessing course content provided by the revising of the Zinsser text, and the number of hours available for lectures in the basic course for medical students have not changed. The flexibility of the third-year elective system and the introduction of integrated departmental and interdepartmental programs represent significant new opportunities for teaching interested students in depth. Even if students do not avail themselves of these further training opportunities, the first year course content, combined with gradual exposure to Microbiology and Immunology within the framework of advanced training in the practice of general medicine, will provide the fund of knowledge necessary for the informed and rational management of infectious diseases and immunologic deficiencies and abnormalities. Our experience is that this approach to medical education is not only highly successful, but meets the wishes and needs of the modern medical student.

IX. Pharmacology

Toshio Narahashi, PH.D.

Introduction

Pharmacology is in a unique position in the sense that it serves as a tight bridge between basic sciences and clinical medicine. It is composed of three basic elements: drugs, their mechanisms of action, and their therapeutic applications. To fully understand drugs, one must have basic knowledge of the chemistry of drugs. To fully understand the mechanisms of action of drugs, including their actions at the target site, distribution, detoxication, and excretion, one must be familiar with the physiology and biochemistry of animals, organs and cells. To comprehend the therapeutic uses of drugs, one must be aware of the nature of the disease in question and the possible side effects of drugs. Although familiarity with the third element, therapeutic applications, is always the primary goal of the course, lack of any of the three aspects distorts medical pharmacology.

First-year pharmacology teaching

Our current efforts to improve the basic pharmacology course have focused on bringing the three aspects described above into harmony in a manner that will enable students to grasp the basic concepts of pharmacology in a limited period of time. Since the course has been revised almost every year, the highlights of the developments rather than details of yearly changes in the course content are described.

A comparison of the time allocated to pharmacology in the traditional and elective curricula is given in Table IX–1. The total hours allocated to the pharmacology course were slightly increased from 110 hours under the pre-1966 curriculum to 121 hours in the post-1966 curriculum. Two major differences are noted. One is the abolition of laboratory exercises and an increase in lecture hours in the new curriculum. The other is the use of the small group conferences in the new curriculum.

Lectures constitute the major part of our first-year pharmacology course. The lecture series is divided into several sections, each coordinated by a

Table IX–1. Time allocated to the basic course in pharmacology

	Traditional curriculum[a] (1964–65) Hrs.	Elective curriculum[b] (1974–75) Hrs.
Lecture	40	61
Laboratory	50	0
Small group conference	0	45
Clinical conference	20	15
Total	110	121

a. Given during the second year.
b. Given during the first year.

single lecturer. The schedule follows the classical format seen in many pharmacology textbooks. Efforts to improve the efficiency and quality of the lectures have included the following:

1. Unnecessary details are eliminated whenever possible within each topic. Since the major objective of the lecture series is to provide students with the basic concepts of pharmacology, too many details impair the lecture by diverting the attention of the students. Even with this effort, at every lecture students are exposed to descriptions of a dozen or more new drugs. It is, therefore, of critical importance that basic principles and concepts be clearly presented as a framework for the integration of this new information.

2. The textbook *Medical Pharmacology*, by A. Goth, has been used for the past several years. This text was chosen on the basis of its conciseness, reasonable comprehensiveness, and the up-to-date information it contains. Notes or syllabi are not used, both because it is difficult to prepare them in a uniform style throughout a course taught by several instructors and also because the lectures and textbook are sufficiently correlated to allow the students to complete the synthesis on their own. *The Pharmacological Basis of Therapeutics*, by L. S. Goodman and A. Gilman, is used as a reference book to provide more detailed information.

3. Although no lecture notes or syllabi are used in the pharmacology course, handouts are occasionally given to the students for use in the lectures. These usually contain tables, graphs, and lists of important drugs and their chemical structures. These data are best handled in this way, rather than through the use of less portable media, such as blackboard or slides, because the number and variety of names of drugs make the subject initially confusing to the students.

4. The importance of maintaining continuity in lecture topics throughout the pharmacology course cannot be overemphasized. When each small section of the course is taught by different instructors in different styles, students easily lose not only orientation but also motivation. Although some

differences in lecture style are unavoidable when several instructors are involved in a course, it is of utmost importance that each instructor communicate with the other about his lecture content in order to maintain this continuity and to avoid unnecessary duplication. For this reason, the total number of lecturers has been reduced to a minimum. In the academic year 1974–75, twelve lecturers covered the major areas of pharmacology, while several other lecturers covered special areas of clinical topics.

5. Since pharmacology is intimately related to subjects covered in other core courses, consideration is given both to the advocate of unnecessary duplication of material and, as is sometimes necessary, to brief review in order to move from material previously covered in other courses toward its pharmacological implications. For example, one full hour is spent at the beginning of the pharmacology course in reviewing the anatomy and physiology of the autonomic nervous system, because without a complete understanding of the system it is impossible to learn its pharmacology. Acid-base balance, cardiac muscle physiology, and other topics are similarly treated.

Small group conferences

Since 1970–71 the pharmacology faculty has placed major emphasis upon the small group conference as a teaching technique. Each instructor supervises the same group of sixteen to eighteen students throughout the entire course. The main purpose of the small group conferences is to discuss the topics that have been presented in the preceding lectures. Each group meets once a week for two to three hours. The method of running the conference differs somewhat among instructors, but the general format may be summarized as follows:

Each lecturer prepares a set of exercise questions (mock examinations) which cover the field of his lectures (e.g. cholinergic drugs, cardiac drugs, etc.). The exercise is in the same format as that of departmental examinations and the National Board Examination. The exercise is given to students in each conference room, and they work on it for thirty minutes or so. Then the instructor goes over each question of the exercise, explaining the basis of the correct answers. Questions asked by students also stimulate discussion, which may extend not only to any problems related to the questions but beyond to related areas as well.

The small group conferences impose a considerable burden on some instructors. Each instructor has to teach every field of pharmacology regardless of his specialty, and he has to spend a fair amount of time in preparation for the conferences. It is difficult for a newcomer to the faculty to run such conferences unless he has a Ph.D. degree in pharmacology. New faculty usually spend one or two years as assistant instructors before taking groups on their own.

In spite of this burden on the instructors, the benefits resulting from the

Table IX–2. Enrollment of the third-year medical students in elective courses in pharmacology

No.	Title	Academic year				
		1970–71	1971–72	1972–73	1973–74	1974–75
PHS-209 (B)	Neuronal Physiology & Pharmacology	—	—	—	—	—
PHS-213 (B)	Cellular and Chemical Pharmacology	—	—	2	—	—
PHS-215 (B)	Topics in Developmental Physiology and Pharmacology	—	—	—	—	—
PHS-219 (B)	Tutorial in Physiology & Pharmacology	1	3	9	2	—
*PHS-225 (B)	An Introduction to Neuronal Physiology and Pharmacology	—	—	—	—	—
PHS-252 (B)	Cellular and Chemical Pharmacology	—	—	—	—	—
PHS-252 (B)	Mammalian Toxicology	—	—	—	—	1
PHS-256 (B)	Human Nutrition	—	—	—	—	16
PHS-330 (B)	Pharmacological Basis of Clinical Medicine	—	12	42	57	53
PHS-331 (B)	Laboratory Methods in Pharmacology	—	1	1	1	0
PHS-334 (B)	Pharmacodynamics	—	—	—	—	2
PHS-372 (B)	Research in Physiology & Pharmacology	1	0	4	2	33
*PHS-386 (B)	Laboratory Methods in Electrophysiology	—	—	—	—	—
PHS-387 (B)	Cardiovascular and Respiratory Physiology and Pharmacology I	24	—	—	—	—
PHS-387 (B)	Respiratory Physiology & Pharmacology I	—	14	—	—	—

Academic Year

No.	Title	1970–71	1971–72	1972–73	1973–74	1974–75
PHS-389 (B)	Cardiovascular and Respiratory Physiology and Pharmacology II	11	—	—	—	—
PHS-389 (B)	Respiratory Physiology & Pharmacology II	—	5	—	—	—
PHS-391 (B)	Neurophysiology and Pharmacology I	6	—	—	—	—
PHS-393 (B)	Integrative and Clinical Neuro-physiology and Pharmacology	3	3	0	2	3
PHS-395 (B)	Biochemical Pharmacology I	16	—	—	—	—
PHS-395 (B)	Biochemical Pharmacology	—	12	—	5	0
PHS-396 (B)	Biochemical Pharmacology II	6	—	—	—	—
PHS-397 (B)	Cellular and Chemical Pharmacology I	1	—	—	—	—
PHS-398 (B)	Cellular and Chemical Pharmacology II	2	—	—	—	—
PHS-401 (B)	Metabolic and Developmental Physiology and Pharmacology	2	1	0	0	0
PHS-407 (B)	Membrane Transport Processes in Physiology and Pharmacology I	—	1	—	—	—
*PHS-416 (B)	Biophysics of Excitable Membranes	—	—	—	—	—
PHS-416 (B)	Neuronal Physiology & Pharmacology	—	—	—	2	2

* New courses to begin in 1975–76

— indicates that the course was not given.

small group conferences far outweigh their disadvantages. In addition to the direct instructional benefit to the students generally, each instructor becomes acquainted with a few students, greatly facilitating communication and evaluation. Additionally, this method presupposes communication among instructors, because each of them has to know the teaching material presented by his peers. All instructors are encouraged to attend all lectures, thus avoiding unnecessary duplication in lecture content while assuring continuity in coverage. The intensity of the small group conferences and the necessity of presenting an integrated lecture series improve faculty morale simply because of the level of commitment to the course which they demand.

Medical pharmacology is incomplete without proper references to therapeutic applications. For this reason, clinical conferences devoted to therapeutic applications of various drugs are given every week. Many of these clinical conferences are presented by members of clinical departments, some of whom have joint appointments in the Department of Pharmacology. It should be emphasized that clinical conferences are not mere case reports. Therapeutic applications of various drugs are discussed from the pharmacological point of view. Emphasis is placed on why any particular drug is most suitable in a given instance, how it should be administered, what side effects are to be expected and why, and how the side effects can be managed. In some clinical conferences, patients are introduced to the students. The instructor asks the patient various questions, and elaborates the case for the use of various drugs in treatment. When patients are not presented, data from current literature and clinical cases are summarized in tables and these figures are given to the students.

Third-year pharmacology teaching

The objective of the third-year pharmacology electives is to provide medical students with the opportunity to explore personal intellectual preferences and expand technical capabilities in this field, particularly with reference to the clinical applications of various drugs. The elective program in pharmacology offers students the opportunity to study the clinical applications of drugs to a degree never possible under the old curriculum, and to gain a solid grounding in the laboratory techniques of pharmacological investigation.

A summary of enrollment in courses offered to third-year medical students during the most recent five-year period is presented in Table IX–2. Some of them deal with both physiological and pharmacological aspects of their subjects, while others are limited strictly to pharmacology. Almost all of the third-year elective courses are offered also to graduate students. A course in the pharmacological basis of clinical medicine, which offers detailed analyses of the mechanisms of action and rationales for use of pharmacological agents in disease states, serves as a bridge between the first-year core course and elective work at higher levels. This course is the most frequent elective choice of medical students; enrollment in others is dictated entirely by individual interests.

Overall, the Department of Pharmacology tries to offer a variety of electives which, considered as a group, include opportunities for the study of pharmacological concepts, therapeutic applications, and research techniques. While the ongoing research activities of department members necessarily shapes the range of these offers their scope is broadened, particularly in the area of research methods, through cooperation with the Wellcome Research Laboratories at the Research Triangle Park, just east of Durham. The freedom to enter fully into this cooperative teaching program is but one evidence of the flexibility of the new curriculum. This flexibility is the major benefit of the elective system for the teaching of pharamacology.

X. Behavioral Sciences

Carl Eisdorfer, M.D., PH.D.

Introduction

The need for a significant and relevant contribution from the behavioral sciences to medical education has been a source of concern to many medical school faculties. Several reports and position papers have been generated, most notably the four-volume study, *Behavioral Science Perspective in Medical Education.*[1] Two other such documents have particular relevance. The Committee on Medical Education of the Group for the Advancement of Psychiatry (GAP) surveyed American and Canadian (four-year) medical schools several years ago and presented the data then available on teaching programs in psychiatry and behavioral sciences in the responding schools. The GAP Committee endorsed the strengthening of behavioral sciences teaching in the medical school, although it did caution against "an over-enthusiastic approach in which fundamental biological material would be lost for the acquisition of social science information."[2] A few years later at the Swampscott Conference, Dr. Cope emphasized the current paucity of behavioral science information being offered in medicine and reported that "medical education lacks a behavioral science serving the needs of psychiatry in the sense that physiology and microbiology, to some extent, serve the need of medicine as a discipline." Cope also feels that the behavior science material being offered by conventional departments of psychiatry in the first two years of medical school is not meaningful and that it "certainly does not have anything more than a religious content."[3]

The goals for the behavioral sciences program at Duke were set to reflect the unique mix of faculty and student interests and to be in harmony with the overall educational objectives of the School. One emphasis was to be upon the important data base that behavioral sciences could provide physicians in all disciplines. A second emphasis was placed upon the particular needs of those physicians in training who were contemplating a career in psychiatry or the neurosciences. The third was to generate interest and growth opportunities for a limited number of students, enabling them to focus their interests upon creative scholarly work in the behavioral sciences as these influence health, disease, and patient care.

It was quite clear that, while the student population was of high intellectual calibre, their interests and background in behavioral sciences were highly variable. The range of their educational experiences was extreme and varied from Masters and Ph.D. level accomplishments to little or no undergraduate work. The typical student had a year of psychology or less (frequently sociology) in his or her undergraduate curriculum.

Structure of the program

The program in the behavioral sciences is necessarily structured by the curriculum pattern described elsewhere in this volume. As a "pre-clinical" or basic science, behavioral science appears in the first-year basic sciences core and again in the third-year elective teaching program of the Medical School.

The first-year course in behavioral sciences, entitled "Human Behavior," consists of sixty hours, of which approximately twenty are devoted to lectures and the remaining forty to two-hour small group sessions. In the lecture series, five members of the faculty representing psychiatry, psychology, sociology, and anthropology collaborate in presenting an introduction to the behavioral sciences by discussing such topics as: the importance of multiple-variable approach to human behavior, basic learning processes, individual patterns of psychodynamics, communication patterns, social roles, and the impact of the family and sub-culture upon the individual. These foci are treated in a developmental, as well as a cross-cultural context. The developmental approach involves an analysis of key variables as these change across the life span. The medical student is presented relevant data in behavioral genetics, early learning and imprinting, and appreciation of early parent-child relationships, variables affecting adolescent behavior, middle adult life and aging. Further, it is made quite clear that certain variables differ according to the culture in which an individual is born, raised, matures and dies. It is also emphasized that such cross-cultural differences are not only applicable in a western versus "exotic" framework but that such differences also apply to regional, ethnic, racial, and temporal contexts, and have relevance to interactions with patients.

Small groups, each led by a physician and a behavioral scientist, attempt to make concrete for the student the material covered in the lectures, to present additional concepts from the leaders' frames of reference, and to give the student an opportunity to gain experience in techniques of acquiring information from interaction with patients and others.

The small groups are designed to reflect issues in the course context as these touch upon human growth, development and behavior. Normal infants, children and their parents, adolescents and aged individuals, as well as patients with a variety of medical problems, are interviewed by the faculty and students, who then discuss these interviews in relation to variables presented in the lecture. The behavioral scientist adds information germane to the discussion to bridge the possible gap between the conceptual and real-world issues. The focus of these sessions is to sensitize the students to change through the life span, to factors mediating adaptation to our environment, to psychological, social and cultural factors in mediating response to health and illness, and to the interaction between somatic and behavioral variables.

As indicated elsewhere, in his second year the student is enrolled in a series of clinical clerkships in the major medical areas. One of these is a seven-week rotation in psychiatry during which the emphasis is on supervised patient responsibility. Didactic lectures and seminars are offered to the student and some of these attempt to give clinical relevance to the behavioral sciences material.

The third-year experience in behavioral sciences is composed of two parts. The student is given an option of registering for any number and combination of nineteen courses in the elective curriculum or of selecting a more intensive tutorial program in the multidepartmental Behavioral Sciences Program (BSP). The elective curriculum is taught by psychologists and sociologists as well as research-oriented psychiatrists. The courses are designed to reflect four principal foci in the behavioral sciences: biological bases of behavior, experimental psychology and psychophysiology, development and personality, and social structure and community organization. They are intended not only for those planning a career in psychiatry, but also for the prospective practitioner in any branch of medicine. Since some courses are offered more than once during the academic year, each student has more than thirty opportunities annually to elect work in behavioral sciences.

No attempt is made to develop any specific requirement for representation within these four areas; rather, the foci are accepted as guidelines for the use of the faculty. Instead of offering a gamut of courses, our instructors are requested to define their course offerings as relevant to these four areas, although specific courses reflect the interests of qualified members of the faculty in the Department of Psychiatry.

The weighting of these courses runs from one through eight units per term. Each term is nine weeks long and the academic schedule is composed of four such terms per calendar year (with each student required to carry a nine-credit load per term).

The Research Preceptorship in Behavioral Sciences represents a significant amplification of the other elective possibilities. A student can elect to take this course in any term for a variable number of units, i.e., one through eight. He is assigned to an individual faculty member by mutual consent and expected to work with this preceptor for at least the specified number of hours. This program enables students to work with one of the behavioral scientists in the department for a brief period in order to develop for himself an understanding of a specific area of investigation, including the methodologic approaches, body of scholarship, and laboratory operations in that sub-field. In addition, the Psychology, Sociology, and Anthropology

Departments are accepting our students in graduate level courses for which they will receive credit in the Medical School.

Behavioral Sciences Study Program

For those students interested in an in-depth experience in behavioral science, the 1969–70 academic year saw the introduction of the Behavioral Sciences Study Program (BSP), a thirty-six unit course of study (nine units per term for the full academic year) and not available for less than eighteen units.

The focus of this program is to enable the student to obtain a better understanding of some of the basic processes underlying human behavior. The year-long intensive experience is designed to familiarize the medical student with significant issues in the behavioral sciences and the method-ology used to investigate such issues. An essential component of the program is an extensive period of study in a laboratory or library research project, and a paper is required for the successful completion of the program.

The basic Behavioral Sciences Study Program (BSP-201) concentrates upon individual behavior, as well as the characteristics of group activity. The focus of the BSP is in one aspect contiguous with, but does not overlap, the Neurosciences Study Program, which focuses primarily upon the inter-cellular and sub-cellular bases of neural response; at the other end the BSP is close to sociologic and anthropologic studies.

In order for the medical student electing for the Behavioral Sciences Study Program in the third year to have the intensive and meaningful experience for which the study programs were developed, it was felt necessary for him to focus on one of the two major sub-divisions which constitute this program.

Option A: One of the sub-divisions is for the student wishing to concen-trate upon processes which take place primarily within the individual or-ganism. Its faculty is oriented toward biological and experimental psy-chology and includes individuals with a background in behavioral genetics, central nervous system effects on behavior, autonomic nervous system reponse to stress and its behavioral correlates, physical anthropology, learn-ing and conditioning, memory, sensation and perception, ethology, and comparative (cross-species) analysis of behavior. The faculty for program A include the following:

Psychiatry Department (Behavioral Sciences)—seven faculty mem-bers*
Pathology Department - three faculty members
Zoology Department - one faculty member
Anatomy - one faculty member

*Also members of the appropriate department in the Graduate School of Arts and Sciences

Physiology - one faculty member
Biomedical Engineering - one faculty member

Option B: For those students wishing to focus their interests upon inter-personal or group behavior or certain aspects of group process, an alterna-tive study plan (Option B) was developed. This option has as its major foci human development, personality and motivation, group processes, and so-cial structure. The faculty have been recruited for their expertise in these areas, including the analysis of small group behavior and family structure. Sociological approaches to human behavior are reflected in the opportunity to investigate community and social organization, population and demo-graphic studies, and medical economics. The faculty representatives outside of the Department of Psychiatry include members of the Graduate School Departments of Psychology, Sociology, Anthropology, and Economics. The faculty for program B with their departmental affiliation include:

Psychiatry Department (Behavioral Sciences)
   A) Sociology—four faculty members*
   B) Medical Psychology—six faculty members*
Psychology Department—three faculty members
Sociology and Anthropology
   A) Sociology—two faculty members
   B) Anthropology—two faculty members
Economics—one faculty member

The student wishing to elect for the BSP in his third year must choose one of the sub-programs in consultation with the program director and members of the staff. The program director and the student set up the program on an individual basis and a preceptor is selected by mutual consent. Each sub-program has a one and one-half hour weekly required seminar, but the great bulk of the student's time is spent in a research preceptorship experience. This is devoted to reading, laboratory experiences, and interaction with the faculty and fellow students in his discipline, and is designed to give him an opportunity to study an area in depth while obtaining a broader base of knowledge in his field. He is expected to work for the academic year with one of the faculty members listed in his program and to produce a paper based upon research in the laboratory or library. Faculty are recruited as voluntary participants in this program. The only incentive for participation has been the excellent quality of the students and what one termed the "ego massage" of working in this perceptorship program.

An upper limit of ten students has been established for such sub-programs in order to ensure close student-faculty interaction. In addition, each student may elect to participate in up to two graduate or medical school courses per semester as deemed advisable after consultation with his preceptor.

The response of the students to this program and the behavioral science

*Also members of the appropriate department in the Graduate School of Arts and Sciences

curriculum in general has been excellent, as evidenced by pre-registration choices. For 1969–70, for example, approximately 8 percent of the rising juniors' preregistration for 1972–73 included seven full-time BSP enrollees (approximately 7 percent of the class) in addition to those in the elective program. Of the seven students now indicating their intention to take the year-long program, only four are definitely planning a career in psychiatry and three have plans for other specialities. One of these is planning for a career in internal medicine, one in pediatrics, and one in public health and international medicine. Student interests seem much more directed toward social and community studies than personality or experimental psychology; these students indicate that an understanding of social processes and community structure is not stressed elsewhere in their training and is their greatest weakness.

Prospects

A significant aspect of this revision in the Medical School curriculum is its implication for postgraduate medical education. The medical school graduate with well-developed basic and clinical science skills in specific disciplines is a challenge to our current residency training programs. At this time, the residency training is predicated on medical generalists whose training and experience are very similar. Psychiatry residency programs have been organized to reflect the paucity of behavioral science and clinical psychiatric information in undergraduate medical education. With a number of medical schools currently proposing or actually operating a revised curriculum, this assumption is no longer valid. The new M.D. with such a good educational experience would be correct in assuming that many aspects of current residency training ignore contemporary curriculum changes. Indeed, many residencies have the traditional, if not rigid, structure which medical schools have already shed.

The need exists to explore the possibility of more flexibility and a greater number of options to be offered the resident as a first step. Modifying certain aspects of residency training in the early years, with rapid acceleration of intensive sub-speciality options and greater investment in the scientific base of medical practice, may result in a better-trained and more valuable specialist than has hitherto been possible.

References

1. A Study for Teaching Behavioral Sciences in School of Medicine. National Center for Health Services Research and Development, Contract No. HSM 110-69-211, 1972.
2. Group for the Advancement of Psychiatry, "The Pre-clinical Teaching of Psychiatry." Vol. 5, Report No. 54, New York, 1962.
3. O. Cope, *Man, Mind and Medicine: The Doctor's Education.* Philadelphia and Toronto: J. B. Lippincott Co., 1968.

Clinical Sciences

XI. Introduction to Clinical Science

Wendell F. Rosse, M.D.

The introduction of students directly to patients and their medical problems is one of the most important aspects of the early medical school curriculum. It is here that each student begins to apply what he has learned in the basic sciences to the understanding and care of patients. It is, further, a time of personal transition since, for the first time, the student must begin to assume the role of physician, and do it convincingly.

In order to begin to understand patients and their problems, the student must learn to gather data about them. Traditionally, three aspects of data-gathering have been taught in introductory courses: history-taking, physical diagnosis and laboratory diagnosis. Both history-taking and physical diagnosis are usually taught as a unit in a course labelled Physical Diagnosis. In this course, students usually are taught how to obtain an autobiographical recounting of events, how to obtain information from other sources, how to organize the information into a coherent history, how to perform a physical examination (with an understanding of the significance of abnormalities in this examination), and how to begin to formulate the information gathered into a coherent outline describing the patient and his problems.

The introduction to the laboratory in the gathering of information about the patient is usually organized into a course variously called Laboratory Medicine, Clinical Pathology or, at Duke under the old curriculum, Clinical Microscopy. In this course, students are usually taught how to do simple laboratory procedures, how to interpret laboratory results, and how to relate these to the problems of the patients.

Under the traditional curriculum, the introduction of the student to the patient and to the methodology of data-gathering was very well provided for, since a large part of the second semester of the Second Year was taken up with Physical Diagnosis and Clinical Microscopy. In the Physical Diagnosis course, a series of didactic lectures were given and, at least twice a week, small groups of four to eight students were taught on the wards by an instructor in the techniques of history-taking and physical diagnosis. A total of 208 hours were spent in these exercises and by the end of that time the students were usually very well prepared for their clinical rotations in the third year.

Clinical Microscopy featured a lengthy set of lectures and a laboratory, held once or twice a week for four hours, devoted to learning very carefully the techniques of simple laboratory examination. These techniques, such as hemoglobin determination, hematocrit determination, reticulocyte count, differential white count and so on were thoroughly taught, since the student was expected to perform these simple laboratory examinations on his own patients during the clinical rotations. In addition, some discussion of the use of other laboratory data in diagnosis of the patient was taken up. A total of 156 hours was spent in this course.

With the coming of the elective curriculum, it became apparent that this leisurely method of teaching would not be possible. The Physical Diagnosis and Clinical Microscopy courses were moved into the first year where, taken together, they occupied about ninety-six hours. Clearly, radical adjustment in teaching techniques had to be made to accommodate this drastic reduction in time allotment.

During 1966–67, the first year of experience with the elective curriculum, the Physical Diagnosis and Clinical Microscopy courses were given throughout the semester, much as they had been under the old. However, under the new format, each course met every other week and, further, the courses were being given at the same time as six or seven other courses in the first year. After this initial experience, which was distressing to students and teachers alike, it became apparent that the course must be concentrated in a shorter time span. Students had difficulty in maintaining continuity when the course was given only once in two weeks and the course got lost amid all the other courses which competed for the student's attention. Therefore, over the next few years, the material introductory to clinical medicine gradually was concentrated into the final six to eight weeks of the first year, when usually only one or two other courses were being given.

We also felt that since both courses essentially involved the teaching of how to obtain data about patients, it would be better if they were amalgamated into a single course to be called Introduction to Clinical Medicine. In this way common planning would permit integration of the teaching so that discussion of the physical diagnostic aspects of certain organ systems occurred at the same time as the laboratory abnormalities associated with malfunction of these organs were discussed. The examinations were devised so as to relate both to physical examination and history-taking and to laboratory diagnosis. The final examination became a single examination and the general format was that of case presentations with questions concerning either physical examination or the laboratory examination being asked.

Even with this new time concentration, there remained some difficulties in presenting the course at the same time as other courses in the first year. When the decision was taken to end the medical school academic year in the middle of May in order to coincide with the university calendar, it became apparent that other plans for Introduction to Clinical Medicine would have to be made. There simply was not enough time for all courses assigned to the freshman year.

There were, in addition, two courses being taught in the second year which did not fit well there: Radiology and Community Health Sciences. Accordingly, plans were made to integrate Radiology, basically another science of data-gathering, with Introduction to Clinical Medicine, and to present this course in an integrated fashion by extending the term for seven weeks. Community Health Science was to be given at the same time.

This amalgamation of the three data-gathering disciplines (history and physical examination, laboratory examination and radiological examination) within a concise time span has been used now for three years and is the most useful arrangement of content and timing yet devised. It has the advantage of permitting the three disciplines to be presented by organ systems (see below) without a great deal of other material at the same time. The timing has the disadvantage of prolonging the freshman year. This has been viewed by some students as a hardship but, in general, the students have enjoyed the material being presented so much that they have willingly prolonged the period of intensive study. A few students feel that enough is enough and put off taking their second-year courses until after taking Introduction to Clinical Medicine in the fall term of their sophomore year. The number of these students, however, has not been large enough to disrupt the scheduling process for the second year overall.

When the elective curriculum was initiated in 1966–67, ways were sought to present the material through the use of audiovisual aids and other teaching devices. However, it became clear that the methodology of teaching the practical aspects of physical examination and laboratory examination could not be markedly altered. Because of the time constraints, the students received a great deal less exposure than they had with the old curriculum in the practical business of taking histories and performing physical and laboratory examinations. There appeared to be no way in which this practical physical diagnosis experience could be particularly enriched except by reducing the size of the groups to four students each, which was done. The emphasis in the laboratory diagnosis portion of the course was gradually shifted away from the practical performance of laboratory tests to a more thorough understanding of the use of laboratory information in conjunction with information obtained on history or physical examination in defining the patient's problems. In part this was possible because the actual performance of the laboratory examinations on the wards was gradually de-emphasized as the professional clinical laboratories of the hospital increasingly undertook these examinations. The students were encouraged to examine the laboratory data available on patients whom they examined during the physical diagnosis exercises, and were in some instances asked to make reports before the group correlating these sets of information.

When the revision of the course to include radiological diagnosis occurred, the course was fully integrated across the lines of the three disciplines being taught. All material relevant to a given organ system was presented at the same time by the three faculties. The amount of time allotted to each faculty for lectures during that time was set according to the importance of that discipline in the gathering of data about that organ. Thus, when the heart was discussed, the Physical Diagnosis faculty and Radiology faculty gave more lectures; when the blood was discussed, the Laboratory Diagnosis faculty had a preponderant role. The total amount of lecture time was stabilized at about ten hours per week.

The laboratory time in the disciplines was adjusted so that each student had eight hours of P.D. experience (two four-hour sessions) and four hours each of L.D. and R.D. experience (two two-hour sessions) each week. The emphasis in the laboratory time for each discipline was integrated with the organ system being reviewed in the lectures.

When the elective curriculum first was introduced, the students were very confused by the welter of material presented to them. The confusion has decreased as the course has been gradually consolidated, amalgamated and integrated. It is unrealistic, however, to suppose that students taught physical diagnosis under the much abbreviated new curriculum would be as adept, when they first entered the ward, as those taught from the old curriculum. They were not, as attested to by the physicians observing the students during their clinical rotations and by the students themselves. It was originally suggested that what was lost of the original Physical Diagnosis and Laboratory Diagnosis sections of the old curriculum could be made up during the second-year rotations under the new curriculum by added emphasis from each of the clinical departments on physical examination in these areas.

Initially this was not successful, at least in the view of the students. They felt that they were not rigorously checked for their physical findings in all instances. The general physical examination was sometimes not the main interest of the clinical instructors (e.g., in Psychiatry or Obstetrics) or the instructors did not have time to review all the physical findings in detail. The students also felt that the time in didactic teaching was being used to teach the specialty involved rather than to teach fundamental physical diagnosis and history taking. Each year, for this reason, the students and a good portion of the faculty suggested that more time be spent in the introduction to physical diagnosis and laboratory diagnosis. Although the revised schedule is more nearly adequate than the original, there is continuing demand for the assignment of more time to observe practice in physical diagnosis.

The history of development of the course from Physical Diagnosis and Clinical Microscopy through Introduction to Clinical Medicine to the present course has shown how revisions must be made continually in order to speak to the problems induced by the adoption of a new curriculum. These revisions have increased the efficiency of use of the more limited time allotted to these disciplines so that students are now sufficiently prepared to continue their learning without special help. They have responded to these revisions with helpful criticisms and have had part in their formulation. Although the program is far better than at the inception of the elective curriculum, further improvements will come from continued thought and receptiveness to change.

XII. Community Health Sciences

E. Harvey Estes, M.D.

The Department of Community Health Sciences did not exist prior to July 1966. There was, however, a tradition of teaching in the area of preventive medicine which extended back to the earliest years of the Duke University Medical Center. Catalogue descriptions show an emphasis upon such public health and sanitation problems as the preservation of sanitary water, milk, and food supplies, as well as the investigation of infectious disease epidemics. Usually the lectures and laboratories covering these areas were conducted by faculty members from several departments, with a major input also from visiting lecturers from the University of North Carolina School of Public Health and from local public health officials. Only from 1938–50 was there a separate Department of Preventive Medicine.

In 1964, departmental status was reestablished, with Dr. David T. Smith as Chairman and Drs. William DeMaria and E. C. Long as faculty members. This group reoriented the teaching program by stressing epidemiologic principles, environmental factors in health and illness, illness and care in the family environment, and international health problems. Elective courses were established in which the student spent one or more summers working in Guatemala, or another similar area, in which epidemiological and preventive medical principles could be demonstrated in a practice setting.

In 1965, prompted by the impending retirement of Dr. David T. Smith, a faculty committee was appointed, chaired by Dr. Roy Parker of the Department of Obstetrics and Gynecology, to study the future role of preventive medicine in the Duke curriculum and to make recommendations regarding the future of the Department of Preventive Medicine. There was a widespread feeling, not only at Duke but also throughout the country, that sanitation and public health topics were no longer worthy of large blocks of curricular time and that most aspects of preventive medicine should be interwoven with pediatrics, internal medicine, psychiatry and other clinical teaching.

The committee concluded that a new Department of Community Health Sciences should be formed. Its focus was envisioned as being considerably broader than that of the Department of Preventive Medicine. It was seen as focusing on teaching the medical student about those problems relating to the organization and delivery of health care (both preventive and remedial) to groups of patients as constrasted to problems presented by an individual patient. These concerns included access to care, cost of care, convenience and dignity of care, and organization and efficiency of care. The new department was seen as utilizing such diverse disciplines as economics, the social sciences, computer science, management science, and others in achieving its goals. The disciplines of biostatistics and epidemiology were also included in its scope.

The Department of Community Health Sciences began operation in July 1966. Its first chairman, Dr. E. H. Estes, Jr., was recruited from the Department of Medicine, and its first faculty were those previously in the Department of Preventive Medicine. Two new faculty members, recently recruited by Preventive Medicine, became the first full-time members appointed in the new Department of Community Health Sciences. These were Dr. Michael O'Fallon (Biostatistics) and Dr. Siegfried Heyden (Epidemiology). The chairman and the remaining faculty were shared with other departments and the Medical School administration.

The courses offered by the new department were a continuation of the courses previously taught in Preventive Medicine. One course, CHS 200, was required of all students. It included lectures in Biostatistics, Epidemiology, Community Health, Industrial Medicine, and the Transmission and Natural History of Disease. Other courses included the elective in "Prospective Medicine," covering human responses to environmental agents, which was taught by Dr. DeMaria. There were two elective courses in International Health, taught by Dr. Long. One of these was a program in which the student spent a portion of time in Guatemala or Nicaragua. There were also electives in Biostatistics, taught by Dr. O'Fallon, and in the Student Health Program, with Dr. Persons and Dr. Portwood as instructors.

As the Department began, it was one of the first such departments in existence in the United States. There were, as a result, very few models which could be used for patterning a program. There were no textbooks, and no journals relating to community health. There was also no training program in this discipline, and no source of previously experienced faculty. The original concept at Duke presupposed that the Department should attempt to provide solutions to some of the major problems facing groups of patients. By learning to solve these problems, a body of information could be accumulated, which could then be imparted to future generations of medical students. The problem of access to medical care was selected as a major problem for solution. The most available methodology for increasing access at that point in time, was to devise methods of increasing the productivity of the individual doctor's office.

This emphasis led to the establishment of two programs very early in the history of the new department. The first of these was an exploration of the use of computer technology in increasing the efficiency of the office practice. The second was the use of new types of health manpower for the same purpose.

The computer program began in 1967, at which time Dr. Howard K.

Thompson joined the Department, soon followed by Dr. W. E. Hammond. These two faculty members began to explore the use of a computer-generated medical history and the value of computer-supported data systems.

The Duke Physician's Assistant Program, which began in the Department of Medicine in 1965, was reassigned to the Department of Community Health Sciences in 1967. This initiated the activities of the Department in exploring the uses of new intermediate levels of health manpower. Experience in the establishment of clinics and new health facilities was added in 1968, when the Department catalyzed the development of a group practice in Durham. This clinic still functions under the name of the Croasdaile Clinic.

In 1969, in an attempt to explore solutions to the problems of "doctorless" communities, the Department established a program in two communities utilizing community health workers recruited from community residents in conjunction with physician's assistants. This was the beginning of an interaction with the Bragtown and Rougemont/Bahama communities of Durham County. This activity eventually led to the establishment of satellite clinics, which have now been absorbed into the Lincoln Community Health Center, located at Lincoln Hospital. The relationship between the Department and these two communities persists, under the direction of Dr. Eva Salber and her staff.

The most recent programmatic development within the Department is represented in the addition of the Family Medicine Program. Throughout the early years of the Department, it was obvious that the public was interested in a more accessible type of medical practitioner, one who was able to offer preventive maintenance, continuity of care, and a correlative function between the patient and his family and a complex medical system.

The Duke faculty did not favor the establishment of a family medicine program when the Department began in 1966, nor was it receptive to a similar proposal in 1970. However, in conjunction with Watts Hospital and with the vigorous support of Dr. Edward Williams, then the Chief of the Medical Service at Watts, plans gradually evolved for a Family Medicine Program as a joint endeavor between the Department and Watts Hospital. In 1972, the first residents were admitted to a Family Medicine Program at Watts Hospital, and Dr. Lyndon Jordan was added to the faculty as the first teacher in the Family Medicine Program. Dr. Jordan chose to return to his practice after one year, but he was followed by Dr. William J. Kane and Dr. Collin Baker, then by several other family physicians. These physician faculty members established an important new teaching setting at Duke in the form of a model office emphasizing the teaching of ambulatory care and continuity of care. The Family Medicine Program has provided a very useful clinical dimension to the activities of the Department, which does not have bed assignments within Duke Hospital. In addition, the Duke medical student is now offered a new and different career role model.

The Department of Community Health Sciences, as it exists in 1975, consists of six divisions. These are: Information Sciences Division (including biostatistics, epidemiology, computer sciences, medical records and records systems), Health Teams Division (including the Physician's Associate Program), Clinic Division (including Student Health Service, Employee Health Service, Faculty Health Service, Occupational Health Program, etc.), Community Health Models Division (including health education, consumer advocacy, community health diagnosis, community health planning), Family Medicine Division, and Education Division (including organization of courses and advice to students). The Department offers some courses that are classified as basic science and some that are classed as clinical experiences. "Basic" electives offered by the Department include such areas as medical use of computers, the history of medicine, systems analysis, biostatistics, medical care insurance, the collection and analysis of survey information, the analysis of health care systems, and general tutorial experiences. The "clinical" courses include studies of health care in Durham County, experiences with an epidemiologic field study in Georgia, the use of computers and patient monitoring, experiences with a community education project, clinical experience in ambulatory clinics, a course in philosophical problems for physicians, a course in rehabilitation medicine, experience with community physicians in their own office environment, experience in the University Health Services Clinic, and a course on environmental pollution. The courses in the history of medicine are the most popular among the basic electives, while the clinical experience with local practitioners is the most frequently chosen clinical course.

Three problems related to the implementation of this new program within the format of the elective curriculum deserve expanded comment. These are, in order, the place of the required course in Community Health Sciences in the core sequence, the problem of classifying electives offered by the Department, and the future of the concept of family medicine.

CHS 200 is a required course which incorporates basic fundamentals of biostatistics, epidemiology, and community health. Although it is a continuation of a course taught, prior to 1966, by the old Department of Preventive Medicine, it has been modified to reflect the broader interests of the new department as described above. The course introduces the student to problems encountered by patients who do not have geographic or economic access to health care, problems faced by physicians who must combine a large patient load with task delegation and management duties, problems of the cost of medical care, ethical issues, etc. Biostatistics and epidemiology were reorganized to emphasize their relevance to medical practice. These changes were apparently well received by students, yet the course suffered from poor attendance and student participation. The nature of this problem is worthy of considerable attention.

Under the traditional curriculum, a lecture-type course in the second year was reasonably well tolerated. Even though not patient-related, the content and the teaching form were consistent with other concurrent courses. Under the elective curriculum, the second-year student was in the midst of his first clinical experience, dealing for the first time with patients, disease states, surgical procedures, etc. These activities were tremendously absorbing and interesting to the student. A lecture or any other activity not directly directed to individual patient care now was viewed as an intrusion on his primary learning process. The student was no longer willing to spend time and energy on topical material which had no obvious relevance to clinical experience or to patient care.

The attitude of the student toward the basic sciences also changed. He now had a sense of which material was relevant and which was not. Material which would have been dutifully absorbed or memorized, on the premise that it must be useful because the instructor was teaching it, was now rejected. This change in student attitude and orientation was reflected throughout the new Duke curriculum, which was generally seen as a drift within basic science courses toward increased numbers of clinical correlations, and increased utilization of clinical teachers in basic science courses, a trend not yet fully understood or accepted. CHS 200, lecture-dependent and not clearly clinical, did not fit.

The course suffered other problems as well. Frequently the house officer on a busy medical floor simply was unwilling to allow a student assigned to his ward to depart to attend a lecture. From his perspective, nothing could possibly exceed in importance the experience immediately at hand on the ward. The clinical chairmen, who agreed with this opinion, were unwilling to insist that the student must be allowed to attend this required teaching exercise. This fact accounted in large part for the poor lecture attendance, and confronted the student with a very frustrating and often impossible choice.

Unhappiness on the part of the students, course instructors, and other clinical departments, eventually led to a change in the time assignment of CHS 200. In 1973, this course was assigned to a time block at the end of the first year, where it shared time with an expanded clinical diagnosis course and a fundamental course in radiology. The new assignment has solved many of the above scheduling problems, and has made the course more acceptable to all. The lessons learned from CHS 200 and its problems, however, remain relevant to all other courses, particularly basic science courses, and should be repeated for emphasis. The intense exposure of a medical student to clinical problem-solving transforms him into a much more discriminating and critical student. He is intolerant of learning "basic" material simply because an instructor has an interest in it, and he must see a reason for his effort. This demands a different skill on the part of the instructor from that which has brought success to the basic scientist in the past. One solution is skillfully to incorporate the clinician into the planning and teaching of the course, to the profit of clinician, basic scientist, and student.

This process is actually a validation of the elective curriculum in that the student changes his choice of material to be learned on the basis of experi-

ence. It demands, however, significant flexibility on the part of the basic
science faculty and resistance to pressures either to return to a rigidly
assigned sequence of courses or to eliminate clinical content on the grounds
that this teaching is less rigorous and not "true science." Another lesson
learned is that didactic background course work, thought to be needed by all
students, yet difficult to relate to individual patient problems, should be
taught prior to the student's first intense patient contact.

A second problem has arisen from the attempt to classify all courses
offered by the medical school as either "basic" or "clinical." This division
was originally made in order to determine the content of the core years and
the scope of choice in the elective years. However, given the trend toward
clinical correlation of basic science material, the current primary separation
is between courses taught by traditional basic science departments and
courses offered by traditional clinical science departments. A new course,
based on a non-traditional disciplinary approach to problem-solving, runs
the significant danger of being accepted by neither established group within
the medical school faculty. A new course, for example, entitled "Economic
Considerations in Health Care," would probably be classified by a clinical
science group as "basic" and by a basic science group as "clinical."

It has not proved possible to draw definitions of these two categories in
such a manner that new perspectives and methodologies can readily be
accommodated within the curriculum structure. The compromise position
which prevails at the present time is that basic science electives in the social
sciences, management sciences, computer sciences, history of medicine,
ethics, etc. can be taught, but a student can elect no more than one semester
equivalent of total credit within these catagories. This can lead the general
student to be very moderate in his election of such courses, utilizing them as
"flavor" for an otherwise traditional assortment of courses. It also works
positive hardship on the few students in each class who hear a different
drummer and wish to concentrate on such courses. These few must,
nevertheless, march to the regular drummer in order to graduate, and the
department must negotiate constantly in order to be able to offer the variety
of courses it feels is necesary. The common conviction of faculty members
that their particular disciplines are fundamental to sound medical education
makes introduction of new approaches difficult.

The problem of relating non-traditional disciplines to basic science electives is matched, on the clinical side, by difficulty in gaining acceptance of
family medicine as a valid medical career choice. Again, this is a problem
which has its origin outside curriculum design per se. Arguments against this
choice have included the assertions that few students have selected family
medicine in the past, that multispecialty group practice may well replace
the solo practitioner, and that the major effort of Duke should go to training medical specialists, researchers, and teachers. Opposing arguments,
equally persuasive at least, are that Americans are demanding more personalized forms of health care delivery, that multispecialty group practice is

ill suited to the needs of small communities, that there have been few role models in medical schools for students interested in family practice to emulate, and that there ought to be no difference in the quality of training provided for physicians, whatever their ultimate career goals.

On balance, the second set of arguments has prevailed at Duke. Student interest in and outside financial support for programs in family medicine are two major reasons for this but, to the credit of the Duke faculty, the Family Medicine Program has achieved increasing support from other departments since its establishment in 1970. Similarly, although there is individual variation, as in all programs, family medicine residents have gained respect from their peers and colleagues and have impressed students with their strong commitment to their chosen discipline, thus providing an important new role model for the Duke medical student.

Since 1966, the Department of Community Health Sciences has grown from nine courses and twelve full- and part-time faculty appointments to twenty-four courses, forty-nine full- and part-time regular faculty appointments and twenty-six additional clinical appointments. These quantitative measures, however, cannot in themselves reflect the quality of the continual interchange—including some conflict—with both basic science and clinical departments, through which a viable program has evolved. Often an agent for change within the Medical Center, both in basic and clinical teaching, the Department of Community Health Sciences is both an expression of the new curriculum and a measure of its ability to adapt to the developing health care needs of Americans.

XIII. Radiology

Richard G. Lester, M.D.

Prior to the inauguration of the elective medical school curriculum, there were no organized educational activities in Radiology for undergraduate medical students. Formal teaching responsibilities for the Radiology faculty were limited to postgraduate (resident level) instructional programs. There were occasional contacts with undergraduates, usually during visits by medical students to the Radiology Department and occasionally on the wards. It was the perception of the Radiology faculty and other faculty members as well that student knowledge of diagnostic radiologic information was relatively meager, and that the understanding of and the skills in diagnostic radiologic techniques were essentially nonexistent. There was no instruction in the area of radiation oncology. Neither was there instruction by members of the faculty of the Department of Radiology in the effects of ionizing radiations on biological systems, in the diagnosis or treatment of radiation injuries, nor in methods of radiation protection.

The Radiology faculty held that at least a portion of this area of knowledge, understanding and skills was appropriate for all physicians and should be a part of the required curriculum while the remainder should be offered among electives open to undergraduates. This was the subject of extensive, lively debate and discussion subsequent to the appointment of a new chairman of the Department of Radiology in June 1965. As a result of these discussions, a compromise solution was arrived at, not entirely to the satisfaction of the radiologists nor to those in other clinical departments naturally intent on protecting their own curriculum time during the required year of clinical instruction. This compromise, subsequently modified, is now the basis of the current instructional program.

The original compromise solution was for a series of weekly two-hour "conferences" (in reality, lectures) throughout the second year. These were devoted to the traditional areas of radiology (diagnostic radiology, therapeutic radiology, nuclear medicine, radiation physics and radiobiology). Although a large majority of the students found these lectures of value and interest, a number of problems soon arose. The formality of the lecture was at considerable variance with the personalized instruction available throughout the rest of the second-year curriculum. More important, many of the students found that they were unable to attend these lectures because of requirements placed on them by members of the other clinical departments.

Interestingly, these demands rarely came directly from senior members of the clinical faculty, but were almost exclusively made by ward interns and residents. The demands were often for what some students identified as "scut work," but there were also requirements for the taking of histories, performance of physical examinations, and other seemingly reasonable work assignments which interfered with this two-hour per week session. Many students volunteered that they felt threatened by the requirements placed on them by house staff officers and were told, or suspected, that their grades would be adversely affected if they went to the radiology lectures. Some of the faculty and many of the house officers on other clinical services felt that this series of weekly lectures, and one other similar series of weekly lectures given by the Department of Community Health Services, significantly interrupted the flow of the instructional efforts of the "major" departments.

Consequently, in 1973, a change in the curriculum was initiated which involved the Radiology Department effort. A period of seven weeks was established at the conclusion of the first year and the required teaching activities of the Radiology Department, the Department of Community Health Sciences and the former course in physical examination and history-taking were concentrated together in that bloc. With some minor modifications, this is the system currently in use. The Radiology component of this course consists of a series of lectures and a series of laboratory demonstrations.

Twenty-five hours are devoted to the lecture series, with as many as three devoted to individual topics of particular importance or complexity. Lecture material is organized according to the structure of the body, with individual presentations on advanced techniques introduced as appropriate. The lecture topics are coordinated with the experience of the students in the course covering physical examination of patients.

The laboratory demonstrations utilize the "Laboratory for Learning" material prepared by the American College of Radiology, supplemented by local material. There are representative roentgenograms from a variety of clinical settings emphasizing basic principles and common clinical situations in diagnostic radiology, supplemented by historical, physical examination and pertinent laboratory findings and by reprints of articles and other literature references. Students are divided into six groups of nineteen each. In the two-hour laboratory sessions, the students study the roentgenograms and other material presented for one hour under the supervision of a resident of radiology. During the second hour there is discussion of the material reviewed with a faculty member of the Department of Radiology. In addition, there are a limited number of laboratory demonstrations devoted to therapeutic radiology and to nuclear medicine. Each student has four laboratory-demonstration hours per week. These also are correlated with the course on physical examination.

Both student and faculty response to this program has been mixed. Students have commented, at times, on the varying quality of the lectures and laboratory instructors. The faculty have been disturbed by the very concentrated nature of this program. There may be as many as four laboratory sessions being taught simultaneously. A high degree of involvement by both faculty and residents is required, at least for a short period of time, in order to serve a large number of students while at the same time carrying on the usual clinical responsibilities incumbent upon department members. Further, the faculty of the department is united in the opinion that assigned teaching time prior to the introduction of the student to the other clinical disciplines is not the appropriate period for instruction in clinical radiology. No students have had any of the required clinical clerkships in medicine, surgery, pediatrics, obstetrics and gynecology, or psychiatry although, it should be noted, they have completed the required course in pathology.

The elective programs in Radiology are concentrated in the fourth elective year. A third-year clerkship was offered in Radiobiology but, as it was rarely selected by students, was withdrawn. The basic radiology clerkship includes observation of and participation in the performance and interpretation of the various routine and special radiologic procedures, with direct correlation of this work to diagnosis and patient care. Departmental conferences and student seminars are required parts of this course. Each student meets with the department's professional advisor prior to beginning the course to work out a program that best meets the student's career interests and current scheduling needs. Within the structure of this single course, the student may choose a broad exposure to the field of radiology or may choose to concentrate in an area of particular interest. Sections participating in the clerkship include General Diagnostic Radiology, GI Radiology, GU Radiology, Nuclear Medicine, Diagnostic Ultrasound, ENT Radiology, Orthopaedic Radiology, and Clinical Radiation Therapy.

Three additional electives are offered. The course in Clinical Radiation Therapy focuses upon the clinical behavior of new patients and is aimed particularly at students entering careers in gynecology, otolaryngology, and general surgery. The courses in Pediatric Radiology and in Neuroradiology concentrate upon the special examinations and procedures peculiar to these fields.

Although the Radiology curriculum has not been an unqualified success from the perspective either of students or faculty, it has represented a giant step forward in the teaching of radiology at Duke Medical School. Every student now has at least some exposure to both basic and applied principles of the various subspecialties in radiology and their application to clinical settings. There is no question that the sophistication of Duke graduates in these areas has been positively influenced by this program. In addition, a significant avenue for in-depth learning has been developed through the elective program. Approximately 25 percent of each student class has elected one or more of the four elective courses.

Long term results of this program are as yet difficult to measure. However, a small but significant number of students have elected to enter careers in radiology and it is believed that this is attributable in part to the under-graduate educational effort. In addition, it is the belief of the faculty that the considerably higher level of sophistication of physicians going into other fields is desirable, indeed essential, in an age of increasing use of ionizing and non-ionizing radiations in the practice of medicine.

XIV. Medicine

James B. Wyngaarden, M.D.

The teaching philosophy of the Department of Medicine has always been to involve the student as an actively participating member of the clinical or research team, with as much direct responsibility as he or she is able to assume. Relatively little use is made of the lecture. Conferences are organized on topics relating to a current patient problem. Clinical learning emphasizes the case-study method, individualized reading, and discussion of the patient with house staff and faculty. The student assumes a large share of responsibility for his own learning. No attempt is made to "cover" medicine. Rather, the student is involved in a representative series of learning experiences in which the acquisition of skills and attitudes is emphasized. Thereafter, the student will spend several years in residency training filling in the blanks in his information about specific diseases, arcane diagnostic tests and minutia of therapeutic regimens. The elective curriculum fits this philosophy better than does the traditional curriculum.

The Department of Medicine participated in all four years of the traditional Duke curriculum. It also does so in the new, but the allocations of time have been substantially altered by the curricular revision.

In 1965–66, for example, faculty members with primary appointments in the Department of Medicine gave occasional lectures in basic science courses during the first three semesters. The department did the bulk of the teaching of physical diagnosis and clinical laboratory diagnosis which occupied 18 percent (275 hours) of the second year. There were obligatory quarters in medicine in both third and fourth years. Third-year students were assigned to a non-private inpatient service at Duke Hospital or the Durham VA Hospital. Fourth-year students were sometimes assigned to these units, but more often to the private medical inpatient unit, which was then entirely a general service (except for Neurology and Dermatology), or to the general medical outpatient department. There was one elective quarter in the fourth year; about one-third of students spent this quarter in the Department of Medicine. A personal estimate prepared in 1972 for other purposes showed that the Department of Medicine was responsible for 19.5 percent of all curricular time during the four years of the old curriculum.

Under the elective curriculum, fewer basic science lectures are given by members of the Department of Medicine during the first year. Our most active participation has been in the courses on medical genetics and physiology. The department continues to provide the bulk of the teaching of physical and laboratory diagnosis (introductory medicine) and does so in an integrated fashion, system by system, with emphasis upon correlations with disease syndromes. Initially this course was offered in time sprinkled throughout the second semester of the first year. Later the time was consolidated near the end of the year. Neither plan worked well; the students were generally under heavy pressure from basic science courses taken concurrently. Furthermore, the allotted time, 102 hours, was too short, and the students entered their major clinical year poorly prepared to assume an active role in the workup and management of patients. The burden of upgrading the students in basic medical skills fell upon the house staff. In 1972 the course in introductory medicine was moved to an additional seven-week extension of the first year, into which first-year courses offered by the faculties of Community Health Sciences, Radiology, and Behavioral Science also were moved. The student, having completed his basic science courses, now could concentrate on transitional courses designed to prepare him for major clinical clerkships. Introductory medicine was assigned more time, 140 hours. Since this change the students have entered the second year adequately prepared for their clinical roles. The house staff is no longer engaged in remedial training.

In the transition from old to new curriculum the basic science departments had a double teaching load one year, the clinical departments the next. Our turn came in 1967–68, when third- and fourth-year students under the old curriculum, and second-year students under the new, were simultaneously present on the wards. That year virtually all medical patients on the 77-bed non-private wards at Duke and the 190-bed wards at the Durham VA Hospital were assigned to students, whereas our standard complement of students allows one-third of patients to be assigned exclusively to the medical intern and resident without the necessity of sharing the learning and management role with a student. It was a rather thin year for the house staff, particularly the interns, who made relatively few bedside presentations that year. Everyone agreed that one such transitional year per decade was enough.

In anticipation of the needs of fourth-year students under the elective curriculum, and in order to provide a more varied experience for our house staff, the Department of Medicine had reorganized its 140-bed private medical service along subspecialty lines in 1966. Faculty members were classified according to major divisional interest and the generalists among us were arbitrarily added to specific subspecialty clusters in order to equalize the average inpatient census. Thereafter, interns were assigned to one of nine subspecialty units on the private side: Cardiology, Dermatology, Endocrinology, Gastroenterology, Hematology, Nephrology, Neurology, Pulmonary Disease, or Rheumatology. Five additional residency positions were created so that interns and students in each of these specialties would have a teaching and supervising resident. Patients were assigned to a sub-specialty service not by diagnosis but according to membership of their private physician, many of whom practiced a mixture of general and specialty medicine. For example, periodic audits disclosed that the endocrine service averaged only 60 percent of patients with primary endocrinologic diagnoses, the cardiology service only 75 percent with primary cardiologic diagnoses.

Each subspecialty organized an in-patient clerkship for fourth-year students, with its own work rounds (students, house staff, private physician), separate teaching rounds, conferences, and seminars. When the fourth-year curriculum became wholly elective in 1966, we were able to offer the student a choice of a clerkship in "Advanced General Medicine" on the non-private wards at Duke or VA Hospitals, a rotation in the general medical clinic at Duke, or a clerkship in a sub-specialty at Duke (often including experience in the ambulatory clinic of that specialty) or in some instances at the VA Hospital (e.g., cardiology). In addition, several one- to three-hour credit courses were offered by the department, e.g., electives in Renal Physiology for clinicians, Electrocardiology, Metabolic and Genetic Diseases. These became popular at once, and have remained so since 1969 when the first students who had progressed entirely under the elective curriculum reached the fourth year. In 1968–69, 39 percent of all fourth-year student credit hours were earned in medicine, in 1969–70 this figure was 47 percent, and in 1970–71 it reached 54 percent. It has hovered about the 55 percent mark since.

One casualty of the elective curriculum has been the general medical clinic student rotation. It is available for as little as one-half day per week or as much as full-time for eight to nine weeks, but there have been only a few subscribers even though the general medical clinics at both Duke and VA Hospitals have been supervised by some of our best teachers who are much sought after by students for inpatient teaching.

For a time we experimented with a fourth-year "early internship." Over a period of three years we allowed one or two students per year to begin regular internship duties in July of their fourth year with a whole year of overlap of student and intern roles, or sometimes in January with six months of overlap. The students were carefully selected, and often were a little older than the average and had already invested extra years in education. Even though the students in question emerged after several years of house staff training as competent physicians, we have given up this approach. The "early-interns" were not ready for the responsibilities of housestaff life. They lacked the maturing and broadening clinical experiences of the fourth year. They knew less medicine. They had to be "carried" by their residents. They displayed inefficiencies and anxieties which seemed greater in general than those observed among interns who had met and mastered a greater number of diverse challenges as students.

Members of the Department of Medicine also play an active role in the third year, the elective basic science year, but they do so indirectly. About 25 percent of our 110-member full-time faculty hold secondary joint appointments in basic science departments. They occupy space built by the Department of Medicine through a combination of dollars generated in clinical activities plus matching funds, and the Department of Medicine is responsible for their salaries. This group is heavily engaged in research and is largely grant supported. Many students elect to work with them in the third year, largely under the aegis of the Study Programs, in most of which our physician-scientists play key roles.

These study programs were introduced as interdepartmental teaching efforts in 1969–70, and grew over the next few years to eight in number. In 1968–69 about 1 percent of all third-year basic science hours were supervised by members of the Department of Medicine in the Medical Research Training Program. In 1969–70 this figure grew to 20 percent and in 1970–71 to 30 percent. All of these course hours appear as basic science credit on the student's record. As further examples of the increase in basic science teaching endeavors assumed by the Department of Medicine under the new curriculum, its members give eighteen of twenty-nine lecture-seminars in third-year clinical pharmacology (1975) and five of eighteen similar offerings in the clinical correlation series in first-year biochemistry. The weight-averaged percentage of all hours of the curriculum now taught by faculty holding primary appointments in and paid by the Department of Medicine was 26 percent in 1970–71. If there has been any recent change, it is in the nature of further increase.

The Department of Medicine is enthusiastic about participating in science teaching. It is worth restating that our members do so under the mechanism of joint appointments in basic science departments, which are awarded on the basis of solid credentials in fundamental research in the discipline, and upon the initiative of the basic science department chairmen. Furthermore, invitations to participate in third-year teaching derive from the basic science departments. This practice places the responsibility for quality control of basic science teaching where it belongs.

The faculty of the Department of Medicine has more than doubled since the key decisions were taken with respect to the elective curriculum. It is difficult to say how many of the new faculty were appointed in response to the increased teaching requirements of the curriculum. No doubt some were, but a more important factor has been the growth of special programs within the department related to increased clinical demands, such as the Coronary Care Units, Respiratory and General Intensive Care Units, the Epilepsy Center, the Cancer Center, Renal Dialysis and Transplant Program, Clinical Pharmacology, the Endoscopy Unit, the Ambulatory Care Center at the V.A. Hospital, greater participation in community-based programs, and expanded research efforts in computerized handling of medical information and in basic pathophysiology of disease.

Evaluation of the consequences of any modification of an educational program is difficult, because the "experiment" cannot be controlled. The faculty becomes more excited and committed to teaching. The faculty-student ratio changes. The quality and character of the student body changes. Societal pressures change and profoundly influence student attitudes and choices.

The students do surprisingly well on the wards in their second year. They master the methods of the medical workup about as well as their earlier third-year counterparts. Bedside presentations, however, seem to go a little more slowly. The students' grasp of pathophysiology and their ability to use basic science knowledge in the interpretation of clinical problems is not as advanced as with former third-year students in this setting. These observations have not surprised me.

The trade-off of two years of faculty-scheduled time for two years of student-selected choices has been decidedly to the advantage of the student. My own analysis is that at least two-thirds of our students are now doing things educationally that would have been impossible under the old curriculum. I find them a very much more exciting student body because they themselves are more excited about learning as an active process in which initiative and participation have rewards. The fourth-year students now teach each other many more things because each has had at least one unique experience. Perhaps somewhat less than one-third of our students achieve approximately the same education they would have acquired before, with little more than a rearranging of sequences of courses. However, I suspect that even these students have gained something special from the experience, because they have now selected these courses for their own reasons.

In addition, our students have moved up several notches in competition for internships throughout the country. The great majority of our students now qualify for highly competitive university-based graduate programs. This by no means indicates that they all enter specialties. A larger proportion of Duke students do enter academic careers than the average nationally, but about 85 percent of our students practice clinical medicine at the completion of their training. I believe that the Duke curriculum constitutes one model of a flexible training program which reduces the compartmentalization between the latter years of medical school training and the early years of graduate training, and allows a larger percentage of students to identify early that area of medicine in which they will be happiest and most productive.

References

1. P. Handler and J. B. Wyngaarden, "The Bio-medical Research Training Program of Duke University." *J. Med. Educ.* 36 (1961): 1587–94.
2. H. O. Sieker, "New Curricular Approaches in Undergraduate Medical Education." *Arth. Rheum.* (1968): 240–45.
3. G. A. Kelly and S. Kizer, "Reactions of Recent Graduates to the New Curriculum at Duke University." In *The Changing Medical Curriculum, Report of a Macy Conference*, ed. V. W. Lippard and E. Purcell. New York: Josiah Macy, Jr., Found., 1972, pp. 175–78.
4. J. B. Wyngaarden, "The Medical Curriculum at Duke University." *Bull. N.Y. Acad. of Med.* 49 (1973): 293–98.

XV. Surgery

David C. Sabiston, Jr., M.D.

With the adoption of the elective curriculum in 1966, the alterations in the surgical curriculum were substantial. All of the required work in surgery is currently given in an eight-week period, thus making it necessary to select critically the topics which are included. The faculty of the Department has chosen to place primary emphasis upon those principles which characterize the discipline of surgery and its specialties.

The core course

The required course in surgery is given in the second year, and emphasis is placed upon those basic principles which form the foundation of surgical diagnosis and treatment. Stress is placed upon those subjects which have their origins in objective laboratory and clinical documentation. These include surgical antisepsis and bacteriology, the management of wounds, inflammation, shock, fluid and electrolyte balance, the metabolic response to trauma, the biology of neoplastic disease including chemotherapy and immunotherapy, gastrointestinal physiology and its derangements, and disorders of blood coagulation, thrombosis and embolism. These subjects are applicable equally to general and cardiothoracic surgery as well as to neurosurgery, orthopaedics, otolaryngology, plastic surgery, and urology.[1] Throughout the course, emphasis is placed upon the most meaningful and lasting form of clinical instruction, that is, individual study of the patient. Each student is assigned patients in rotation, and each case is reviewed in detail with members of the resident and senior staff. Maximal student participation is sought in the establishment of the diagnosis and planning of therapy in all patients.

The primary goals of the Required Course in Surgery are to acquaint the student with the basic principles in surgery and to provide a basis for application in actual practice. Primary emphasis is placed upon study of each patient, and this experience is supplemented by a series of informal seminars. It is intended that the course provide a basic foundation in surgery and prepare the students for a wide variety of elective courses in surgery and the surgical specialties available in their fourth year. A block schedule showing daily assignments is depicted in Table XV–1.

The students are divided into equal groups with ten to twelve in each, one

XV-1. Department of surgery: required course in surgery—second year

Monday	Tuesday	Wednesday	Thursday	Friday	Saturday
7:00–8:00 Resident rounds	7:00–8:00 Resident rounds	7:00–8:00 Resident rounds	7:00–8:00 Resident rounds	7:00–8:00 Resident rounds	Surgical grand rounds 7:30–9:30
	Teaching rounds 8:00–9:30		Teaching rounds 8:00–9:30		Teaching rounds 9:30–11:00

Work with patients, general operating rooms, reference reading

Monday	Tuesday	Wednesday	Thursday	Friday
Surgical seminar 1:00 – 3:00	Surgical seminar 1:00 – 3:00		Dr. Sabiston's conference 2:00 – 3:00	Surgical seminar 1:00 – 3:00
Surg. specialty demonstration 3:00 – 4:00	Surg. specialty demonstration 3:00 – 4:00		Surg. specialty demonstration 3:00 – 4:00	Surg. specialty demonstration 3:00 – 4:00
	Surgical staff conference 4:00 – 5:30			Combined cardiac conference 4:00 – 5:30

group being assigned to the service at the Duke Hospital and the other to the Veterans Hospital. In each hospital, the Chief Resident is responsible for the distribution of patients on a posted roster with planning to assure maximal variety in types of clinical disorders. All students are assigned to a resident team with the intention of providing the student maximal participation in patient care. The history and physical examination as recorded by the student are carefully reviewed and annotated by the particular resident. The student is encouraged to participate actively in diagnosis and treatment. The changing of dressings, removal of sutures, care of drains, insertion of nasogastric tubes, administration of intravenous fluids, thoracenteses, spinal puncture, and similar procedures are performed by students under the supervision of the resident and senior staff.

In the past it has been difficult to have an instructor continuously available for the students on the surgery rotation, since the operating room requires nearly every surgeon's presence sometime during the day and often for prolonged periods. In order to alleviate the problem, a resident is assigned each term with the sole responsibility of teaching. This resident is available throughout the day to assist in any manner desired by the students. Specifically, the Teaching Resident reviews the history and physical examination of each patient assigned on an appointment basis with each student. This provides a continuing basis for teaching. This resident also conducts teaching sessions with the students concerning the practical aspects of pre- and postoperative care and is available for instruction and assistance in the care of wounds, drains, thoracenteses, intubations, and related subjects. The students have found the Teaching Resident to be a very valuable and in fact an essential part of the teaching team. Moreover, it has been gratifying to note the response of the Teaching Residents, as this rotation is considered a very desirable one, by their own assessment.

Each group of students is assigned two members of the senior surgical faculty who make bedside rounds for an hour and a half on three mornings weekly throughout the course. At these rounds, the Teaching Resident selects patients for presentation, and the student presents from memory the history, physical findings, and laboratory data. It is considered essential that the student learn from the beginning the significance of committing to memory all pertinent data about each patient in order that it be instantaneously available, as for example in an emergency situation, without need to consult the chart. Thus, on ward rounds each student is expected to be sufficiently prepared at all times to present, from memory alone, patients assigned them. The instructor generally asks questions concerning the patients with queries directed to all students in the group and especially to the students assigned to the patient. He then proceeds to present a rather complete discussion of the specific illness.

While the broad principles of surgery are emphasized during informal seminars three times each week, at the bedside ward rounds the diagnosis and management of specific surgical problems such as acute appendicitis, intestinal obstruction, carcinoma of the breast, empyema, peripheral arterial insufficiency, cardiac defects, pancreatitis, etc. are discussed in detail. Since ward rounds are conducted three days each week and two patients are presented each morning, it is possible to discuss some fifty specific surgical entities during the course. Provision is made to present different disorders on these rounds in order to prevent repetition.

The students meet each morning with the Teaching Resident to discuss specific patient diagnoses and management problems. In these sessions the students have a daily opportunity to ask specific questions regarding details of diagnostic tests, use and dosages of drugs, wound management and other details of management.

Three times weekly a two-hour seminar is held in which the topics of broad relevance to surgery are discussed. Presentations of these topics are made by members of the faculty most closely associated with the subject. In most instances, the instructors have pursued the subject both in the experimental laboratory and in the clinical situation and are recognized for their contributions in the field.

The format of these seminars is arranged such that the instructor presents the subject in the first hour, often with the use of appropriate visual aids. After a ten-minute coffee break, the session continues with the remainder being devoted to student participation as a dialogue. The student is prepared in advance for the session by means of a reading list with several suggested references for each seminar. Each student is asked to be prepared sufficiently to make the seminars a stimulating exchange of ideas.

It is apparent that in the eight-week period assigned to the Department of Surgery for its required course it is not possible to cover thoroughly each of the specialties in surgery. Nevertheless, the surgical faculty agreed that it would be unwise for students to graduate from medical school without having been exposed in some way to such important areas of surgery as neurosurgery, orthopaedics, otolaryngology, plastic surgery, and urology. In the structure of the required course, the chiefs of the respective disciplines provide a demonstration, given as a one-hour session each day for a week for each specialty. In these sessions, the student is provided an opportunity to understand the basis of each specialty together with a concept of its scope with specific patient examples.

Our concepts of the relationship of instruction of students to subsequent residency training in surgery have been previously published.[2] The faculty in each of the surgical specialties places considerable care in the preparation of these sessions. Since it is possible that a student might graduate from medical school without electing further experience in one or more of these surgical disciplines, attendance at these sessions is mandatory. The demonstrations are given daily, are one hour in length, and each of the surgical specialties is assigned one week during the course. Because of the broad scope of these sessions, the surgical faculty feels that the students are more apt to obtain a better experience if the material presented in these sessions is not included in

Table XV-2. Electives in surgery taken by medical students 1967–74

		1967–68		1968–69		1969–70		1970–71		1971–72		1972–73		1973–74	
		E	W	E	W	E	W	E	W	E	W	E	W	E	W
201	Advanced Surgery - Emphasis Cancer			3	26	5	35	5	39	1	2	3	14	2	4
202	Adv. Sur. - Emphasis Cardiovascular-Thoracic							3	8	6	33	5	26	5	10
203	Adv. Sur. - Emphasis Transplantation			1	8					1	2			1	8
204	Adv. Sur. - Emp. Gastrointestinal & Trauma							3	11	2	4				
205	Adv. Sur. - Emphasis Pediatric Surgery							2	13	10	56	2	10		
206	Surgical Aspects of Thoracic Disorders			4	24					1	6				
207	Surgical Cardiology					1	8								
208	Rehabilitation Medicine					3	4								
213	Homotransplantation of Organs			3	6	3	6								
215	Surgical Disease of Blood Vessels & Lymphatics	5	9	13	13	5	5								
217	Surgery of Trauma			11	48	5	20								
219	Advanced General & Thoracic Surgery	8	37	3	21	7	56	8	53	6	44	7	56	4	32
221	Surgical Spec. & Ophthalmology			4	12	3	24	7	51	4	32	4	32		
222	Clinical Dentistry											3	3	2	2
223	Medical and Surgical Renal Disease			10	80	8	60	6	44	1	9	4	32	2	16
225	Investigative Urology			1	8										
227	Clinical Urologic Survey	1	20	3	20										
229	Seminar in Urologic Diseases	1	9	6	6	3	24	2	8			1	3	1	4
230	Seminar in Urologic Diseases and Techniques	3	6	24	48	25	50	21	42	10	20	13	25	31	62
231	Uroradiographic Diagnosis	2	3	3	3										
233	Basic Neurosurgery Course	3	32	20	20	13	23	17	17	10	10	5	5	12	12
235	Clinical Neurosurgery	9	24	3	24	1	8	1	4	4	32			4	28
239	Clinical Otolaryngology	5	12	2	12	7	32	4	16	5	21	7	22	15	51
240	Otolaryngologic Seminar			10	10	12	12	10	10	10	10	12	12	11	11
245	Reconstructive Plastic Surgery	2	18	3	18	3	15					1	6	1	6
248	Invest. & Clin. Approach to Wound Healing Including Tissue Preserv. Mic. of Burns			1	6										

		1967–68		1968–69		1969–70		1970–71		1971–72		1972–73		1973–74	
		E	W	E	W	E	W	E	W	E	W	E	W	E	W
250	Clinical Acute Respiratory Physiology			1	2	6	12	4	8	5	10				
252	Clinical Anesthesiology	5	32	4	32	1	4			4	24				
253	Anesthesiology Research							2	4						
255	Medical Speech Pathology													2	12
257	Med. Spch. Pth. Applied to Reconstructive Plastic Surgery			1	1										
259	General Principles of Orthopaedics	7	56	7	56	5	40	3	17	10	61	17	72	12	58
261	Office and Ambulatory Orthopaedics											1	4		
263	Orthopaedics in the Community Hospital			2	8			1	8	1	4				
267	Clinical Conference in Cerebral Palsy														
273	Athletic Med. - Physical Conditioning & Management of Injuries	1	8	1	8										
275	Electromyography			1	2	1	2	1	2			1	2	1	2
277	Orthopaedic Research					4	6	1	5			1	4		
281	Intro to Fractures & Musculoskeletal Trauma	1	15	5	15	2	6	5	15	9	27	9	27	8	24
283	Orthopaedics of Infants, Children & Adol.	1	16	2	16	1	8	2	12	2	12				
285	Adv. Sur. General and Thoracic					8	64								
291	Cancer: CHS, MED, MIC, OBG, PTH, RAD, & SUR Aspects							6	32	6	32	3	11	5	17
295	Investigative Surgery									1	5				
299	Advanced Surgical Clerkship	4										17	106	16	116
301	Emergency Surgical Care													21	54
700	Early Surgery Internship							2	36	10	102	6	54	6	54
	Total	59	353	151	547	133	530	116	455	119	558	122	528	162	573

E=enrollment
W=weight

the final oral and written examinations in the course. Experience has shown that these sessions are both well attended and well received. Moreover, each of these disciplines attracts significant numbers of students into electives in the fourth year and subsequently into their respective residency programs.

Each week a surgical staff conference is held, during which the two most interesting patients in the hospital at the time are presented with a planned discussion by various members of the staff not only in the Department of Surgery but throughout the Medical Center. After each presentation adequate time is allowed for discussion and the students are encouraged to participate in these sessions.

Each week the deaths and complications which have occurred in the Department are reviewed. A member of the staff of the Department of Pathology is present to discuss the postmortem findings, and a thoroughly critical presentation of each case is made. The intent of these sessions first is to establish clearly the cause of death or complication, and then to decide if an alternate approach might have been preferable. Every attempt is made to emphasize possible prevention of complications or death, especially as might relate to future similar cases. A critical analysis of each death and complication on the service is an unusually meaningful teaching experience, and the students find this conference to be both informative and challenging.

On alternate weeks various members of the Department, and at times guest speakers, present research work in progress. These are important sessions to the student as he obtains an understanding of current laboratory investigation. The resident staff contributes original work, and student participation has been open and helpful. The students attend grand rounds each Saturday morning, a two-hour session of clinical presentations with brief, concise remarks being made by the faculty on a number of interesting patients. This is a popular conference and is well attended by students and residents.

At the end of the course, an objective, multiple-choice written examination with 100 questions is given. The more important features of this examination are: (1) the examination is prepared solely from material covered with the students in the course, i.e., the seminars, conferences, and ward rounds, and (2) since it is recognized that students may at times wish to be present in the operating room, causing conflicts with rounds or seminars, any five questions on the examination can be omitted.

An oral examination also is given by a member of the faculty at the end of the course. Each student provides the examiner a list of patients assigned during the course with the appropriate diagnoses, and the oral examination is taken solely from the disorders on the list.

Elective courses

Following completion of the core course in the second year, students are eligible to select from among some thirty-odd elective courses offered in general surgery and the surgical specialties. A list and summary of enrollment in these courses is presented in Table XV –2. In most of these courses, emphasis is placed upon the student's being delegated considerable responsibilities in patient management. In view of the fact that medical students are better prepared on entry into medical school today than before, and maintain this superiority as the course progresses, fourth-year students are now found to perform at a level formerly achieved by interns. In other words, the senior student functions largely as an intern, which is an actual experience since the internship is no longer offered in the Department and appointments are made upon graduation from medical school directly to the first year of surgical residency. Experience has shown that this has been a fully justified move.

In addition to clinical responsibilities, a series of advanced seminars for senior students is designed appropriate for the course. Generally, three seminars are given weekly with advance reference reading assigned for informal discussion with a member of this faculty. Particular stress is placed upon the prerogative of each student to arrange with the Department Chairman or Division Chief any course he may desire which is not specifically listed in the catalog. A number of students utilize this approach in curricular planning, and the surgical faculty has been quite pleased with this flexible approach.

A considerable increase in faculty time has been found necessary in the elective curriculum, as compared with the traditional. Formerly, a number of subjects were presented in sessions for the entire class. In addition, a number of new sessions and clinical rounds have been created involving small groups. Moreover, nearly all of the electives contain only a few students, and a single student often takes an elective as the only member of the course. Thus, individualized teaching has become much more common today than previously.

In considering the problems and difficulties which introduction of the elective curriculum has reduced or eliminated, one could cite the fact that former problems associated with impersonal and whole-class exercises have been eliminated. This has clearly been a positive feature, both for the students and faculty. Moreover, it has allowed them to become considerably better acquainted, and exchange of information is now much more frequently on a personal basis. The primary problem which has been introduced by the elective curriculum relates to the increased time demands imposed upon the faculty to teach relatively small groups. This also requires considerable repetition of discussion of the same subjects, but in general this has been quite well tolerated by the faculty. Generally, those instructors who enjoy teaching draw the larger numbers of students into their elective courses. Overall, the faculty has been quite pleased with the elective curriculum and strongly endorses it.

Reference

1. W. G. Anlyan and D. C. Sabiston, Jr., "A New Approach to Medical Education."
   Surgery 62 (1967): 134.
2. D. C. Sabiston, Jr., "A Continuum in Surgical Education." *Surgery* 66 (1969):1.

XVI. Obstetrics and Gynecology

Roy T. Parker, M.D.

During the early 1960's members of the medical faculty shared two concerns; that the traditional medical curriculum did not provide students with sufficient freedom and opportunity to explore new developments and alternative careers and that, as a consequence, medicine might lose excellent undergraduate scholars to other scientific fields. Simultaneously, movements dedicated to improving the status of women in American society won a widening audience, particularly among students concerned about sex education, sexual freedom without preparation, unwanted pregnancies, criminal abortion, malnutrition, population dynamics, and the availability of adequate health care for the poor. This combination of pedagogical and social pressures broadened the discussion of a new curriculum among members of the Department of Obstetrics and Gynecology into a total reexamination of departmental objectives. The major result was a statement of ten-year goals for the department, set as follows: (1) to establish reproductive biology as the basic scientific orientation of the Department, and to create within it a center of research in reproduction; (2) to redesign the curriculum so as to provide a core experience for second-year medical students plus senior electives appropriate for students not intending careers in obstetrics and gynecology, a core curriculum for residents in obstetrics and gynecology based upon four years rather than five, elimination of the internship as a prerequisite for residency training, and for all students, an experience focused upon outpatient medicine; (3) to develop a Woman's Clinic where the distinction between private and public patients would be eliminated, with care for all provided by practice teams composed of faculty, fellows, residents, students, nurses, and physician associates; (4) to develop explicit standards for female health care; (5) to increase the attractiveness of the residency program, and thereby the effectiveness of departmental teaching, by providing programs leading to certification for three categories of residents: the general obstetrician and gynecologist, the intradisciplinary specialist, and the academic gynecologist; (6) to further improve departmental teaching programs through the development of Fellowships in intradisciplinary Divisions of Endocrinology, Oncology, Perinatology, Gynecology, and Community Health; and (7) to support community health through regional medical programs and annual seminars for the continuing self-education of practicing physicians.

Specific discussion of the undergraduate curriculum must be set in the context of these general purposes. To meet the first objective and to cope with an increasing patient load, two reproductive physiologists, one neuro-endocrine anatomist, one microbiologist, and physicians with specialty training in genetics, endocrinology, oncology, perinatology, gynecology and immunology were appointed to the department. In 1967 new clinical facilities, a combined delivery suite, a medical-fetal research center and a departmental library-conference center opened. The creation of a Division of Perinatology marked cooperation with the Department of Pediatrics, in patient care, teaching, and research in the areas of perinatal mortality and morbidity. Attempting to meet the ethical imperative underlying the fourth goal has reinforced the effort necessary to devise instructional materials which compensate, in increased clarity and effectiveness, for the loss of required teaching time and a reduction in introductory work experience. The mixing of private and public patients in the Woman's Clinic, established in 1974, has won the approval of socially concerned students and has facilitated team approaches to instruction that have benefitted medical students at all levels.

These initiatives shape the experience of the undergraduate students in the Department. The first-year student receives instruction in the fundamentals of obstetric and gynecologic history and pelvic examination during the Introduction to Clinical Medicine course which marks the transition from first- to second-year instruction. Initially, the time devoted to obstetrics and gynecology included four hours of lecture and eight hours of ward experience. Now, however, the lectures are optional, and there is evidence that not all students spend the full eight hours on the obstetrical and gynecologic wards. Since the original allocation of time was not considered fully adequate, the Department developed self-instructional materials which have helped the students to master basic information but which may also encourage them not to use what time is available on the wards to full advantage. Improvement of this experience could help to reduce the difficulties which second-year students encounter in their first ward rotations.

In the second year, OBG-202 is required of all students, and consists of eight weeks in general obstetrics and gynecology. Students attend lectures, work daily in general and special outpatient clinics, and are assigned patients on the obstetric and gynecologic wards. Students share in patient care, teaching exercises, gynecologic-pathology conferences, endocrine conferences, and correlative seminars, and lectures are included.

Performance by faculty and students has improved yearly under the elective curriculum. The second-year clinical program has worked much better since the duration was extended to eight weeks. Beginning in 1964, short clinical rotations at Watts Hospital and Lincoln Hospital (Durham community hospitals) and in six decentralized clinics in northeastern North Carolina counties have provided the students with a community medical experience. Each year the students have praised this outlying clinic experience; its success has been credited to the primary care responsibility given to the students and to the one-to-one relationship of student to resident as they make the trips in the Department station wagon and practice medicine together. The paramedical personnel in the County Prenatal Clinics and Family Planning Clinics have been highly supportive of students and residents, and both groups respond extremely well to being treated as primary physicians. In contrast, the students have been constructively critical of their experience in the Duke Clinics. They have complained of long waiting periods for staff consultation, impersonal patient care, and lack of teaching in the clinic setting by residents and faculty. In large measure the fault here lies in the very large number of patients seen daily in the Duke Clinics.

Adaptation based upon experience with the elective curriculum came soon after its institution in 1966. The faculty learned to appreciate that students entering clinical medicine after one year in medical school required more preparation for clinical work than did those students who had maturing time and a two-year preparation for patient problems. This was particularly true for students in the first two or three clinical rotations each year. Most students needed: (1) to review the anatomy and physiology of the female reproductive system; (2) to be introduced to the patient and her problems gradually by seeing fewer patients and spending more time on thorough general evaluations of each one; (3) to develop attitudinal changes that would allow professionalization of the student in regard to his (her) ability to evaluate the female without distracting personal reactions in history-taking and examination (embarrassment, hostility, rejection, disrespect, or enticement); (4) to allow time for desensitization in matters of life and death. The increasing number of female medical students and residents who have made obstetrics and gynecology their career choice have made major contributions toward shaping the response of the Department to the changing roles of women in society.

For third-year electives, the Department has recommended in-depth study in basic science through courses and programs that permit the students to explore their intellectual preferences in keeping with their capabilities. If a student makes an early career decision for obstetrics and gynecology, we advise the study program in Endocrinology and Reproductive Biology. This is an interdepartmental program designed to provide third-year medical students with an opportunity for intensive study in areas of basic endocrinology, neuroendocrinology and reproductive systems in normal and diseased states. Independent study under a faculty preceptor is encouraged. All members of the programs, including faculty, meet weekly for seminars, discussions, and lectures by guest specialists. The student spends four terms in the program. Five faculty from our department (two M.D.'s and three Ph.D.'s) participate in the program along with members of Physiology and Anatomy. As an alternative, we have recommended the Development and Differentiation Study Program. This multidisciplinary program emphasizes molecular, biochemical, cellular, and genetic approaches to the analysis of differentiation and development. Recent concepts in fetal, neonatal, and oncogenic mechanisms and the processes involved in aging and cell death are also explored. This program requires four terms.

Despite faculty consensus that these two study programs are best suited for an in-depth basic science preparation for our discipline, most students have elected a third-year admixture of pathology, microbiology, and other clinically oriented basic science electives. These broadly based third-year electives, chosen on an individual basis, also have proved to be good preparation for careers in obstetrics and gynecology.

For the fourth year, the faculty of our department have developed elective courses primarily for those students who are not planning a career in obstetrics and gynecology but who wish additional preparation in the field. Table XVI–1 describes the range of courses and number of elective opportunities offered each year, while Table XVI–2 presents a summary of our enrollment experience.

Table XVI–1. Elective courses in obstetrics and gynecology

Course	Weight	Terms	Title
OBG-205(C)	4,8	All	Gynecologic Cancer
OBG-207(C)	1,2	All	Pathology: Obstetrical and Gynecological
OBG-211(C)	8	All	Preparation for Practice
OBG-215(C)	4	1,2,3,4	The Infertile Couple
OBG-229(C)	1	1,2,3,4	Endocrinology Seminar
OBG-231(C)	4	All	Basic and Clinical Reproductive Endocrinology
OBG-235(C)	3	1,2,3,4	Cytogenetics
OBG-239(C)	8	All	Perinatal Medicine
OBG-241(C)	4	All	Family Life Sciences
OBG-243(C)	3	1,2,3,4	Sex Education
OBG-245(C)	4 or 8	All	Office Gynecology
OBG-247(C)	4 or 8	All	Clinical Obstetrics
OBT-249	4 or 8	All	Clinical Gynecology
OBG-251(C)	8	All	Advanced Reproductive Endocrinology

The data in these tables indicate that each year approximately 20 to 30 percent of students return for additional study and that most teaching is preceptorial. In the first years of the elective curriculum, the most popular of the courses focusing directly upon practice was OBG-211, Preparation for Practice. In the last two years it has been replaced as the course most frequently chosen by OBG-245, Office Gynecology. The Endocrinology Seminar has been the most popular among the other courses. All courses listed have been taught. The students work as externs on the respective services and have appreciated the one-to-one learning experience with the staff.

For the student who is uncertain of his career choice but thinks that he may

Table XVI–2. Enrollment in electives in obstetrics and gynecology

Year	Number of courses	Students enrolled	Total course weights[a]
1968	18	29	74
1969	13	31	122
1970	13	25	88
1971	19	36	129
1972	15	16	75
1973	24	31	95
1974	25	46	143

a. A student normally enrolls for eight units of course weight per term.

have a major interest in obstetrics and gynecology, we have advised Preparation for Practice (OBG-211(C)). This provides nine weeks of exposure in obstetrics and gynecology in the senior year, or if feasible in the junior year. If he decides at this point that he wants a career in obstetrics and gynecology the remainder of his senior electives are programmed in general medicine, neonatology and courses which shore up his base for primary care.

For the student who has chosen a career in obstetrics and gynecology, and who has a special interest in the medical aspects of our discipline, the following sample schedule is representative:

Course	Weight	Title
Med-207(C)	8	Advanced General Medicine
OPH-205(C)	1	Medical Opthalmology
MED-242(C)	8	Clinical Cardiology
ANE-250(C)	2	Clinical Acute Respiratory Physiology
Peds-225(C)	8	Neonatology
Med-229(C)	8	Nephrology
Surg-230(C)	2	Seminar in Urologic Disease

For the student who has chosen a career in obstetrics and gynecology and who has a special interest in oncology and the surgical aspects of the discipline, the following schedule might be proposed:

Course	Weight	Title
Med-207(C)	8	Advanced General Medicine
Surg-223(C)	8	Medical and Surgical Renal Disease
ANE-250(C)	2	Clinical Acute Respiratory Physiology
Surg-204(C)	8	Advanced Surgery
RAD-215(C)	8	Clinical Radiation Therapy
OBG-207(C)	2	Obstetrical and Gynecological Pathology

We have found that many senior students choose clinical electives to meet their needs only after talking with fellow students. "Word of mouth" is a greater influence among fourth-year students than is faculty advice. In order to avoid overcrowding in some septa, it is necessary to set limitations and demand equal distributions throughout the year. A more disappointing aspect of the senior elective program is that pressure occasionally has been applied to students by some teachers to take certain electives in order to qualify for an internship in the same department. This denies the intent of the elective curriculum to provide collateral work prior to internship and raises again the legitimate question of how departments should spend their senior elective time—broadly, for the benefit of all students, or narrowly, in the training of specialists for their respective fields.

Graduate and residency education

In order to blend graduate and residency education, the internship was made optional for Duke students in Obstetrics and Gynecology beginning in 1967. The residency program was reduced from five years to four and all Fellowships moved to the end of the residency period. This allowed for a continuum from the third year of medical school through the four years of residency. It also reduced the time of preparation for the practice of obstetrics and gynecology to a minimum of four years after graduation. The shorter program also is offered to students from other schools seeking residency.

Fellowship Programs are offered in Perinatology, Endocrinology and Oncology. The Fellowships come at the end of a four-year residency, are of two years duration, and are planned to meet the credentials of the intradisciplinary boards. The Fellows are chosen to qualify as junior faculty members. The "Faculty Fellows" have added significant strength to the departmental educational and research programs. The students appreciate the Fellows as teachers.

For the future

Although we have full data only for those students who choose careers in obstetrics and gynecology, all available evidence suggests that Duke students compare favorably with students of similar academic standing from institutions using more traditional curricula, whether judged by scores on National Board Examinations or on the Annual National Obstetrical and Gynecological Residents' In-Service Examination. This, coupled with enthusiastic student response to departmental teaching, encourages us for the future. Our primary focus will be upon development of the Woman's Clinic as a strong educational primary care unit linked to comprehensive care facilities. All patients are private patients, and are part of the educational program in completely coordinated outpatient and inpatient services. The team practice approach to education, which involves faculty, fellows, residents, students, nurses, and physician associates, offers us the best vehicle for creating, in the busy setting of a medical center, the same enthusiasm for the role of the physician engendered in the more manageable setting of the community hospital. Elective choice becomes the continuing basis for channeling that enthusiasm toward defined career goals.

XVII. Pediatrics

Deborah W. Kredich, M.D.

Samuel L. Katz, M.D.

The restructuring of the Duke curriculum in the 1960's came at a time when educators in pediatrics were discussing the need to change the emphasis of both undergraduate and graduate pediatrics teaching. Traditionally, the discipline was based upon developmental biology and clinical medicine, with particular emphasis upon preventive medicine and general health supervision. Teaching focused on the need for integration of the medical, social, educational and psychological aspects of the patient's development. Gradually, however, the locus of pediatric practice had shifted from the hospital to the ambulatory clinic as the control of infectious diseases with immunization and antibiotics and the improvements in transportation produced a marked decline in the hospitalization of children and adolescents.

A second development which neonatal pediatrics was then experiencing was the revolution in technical support for the life maintenance of newborn infants who were grossly immature or distressed. The construction in medical centers of regional, referral, intensive-care nurseries provided a second teaching laboratory essential to understanding modern pediatrics. Here, however, the crisis nature of decision-making made the involvement of undergraduate students at responsible levels difficult because moment-to-moment assessment of human physiology often was essential to the survival of the patient.

Prior to 1966 most medical students at Duke spent eleven weeks, or one quarter, of their fourth year in a pediatrics clerkship. In addition to experience with hospitalized children, newborns, and clinic patients, each student was required to prepare a major paper on a subject related to one of the disorders encountered among his patients. With the change to a curriculum which brought every student to the Department of Pediatrics in the second year for a seven-or eight-week clerkship, both the goals and the logistics of the course required change.

In the first two years of transition, change took place in conditions of severe overcrowding and a shortage of teaching faculty. Twice the normal number of students had to be accommodated in required clerkships (see Table XVII–1) with no accompanying addition of either faculty or teaching space. As anticipated, students entering the first clerkships of the second year needed considerable basic orientation to hospital and clinic function, physical diagnosis, and patient interview techniques, particularly since the preparatory physical diagnosis course included only one session devoted specifically to pediatrics. During those first two years a "buddy system" was established whereby the fourth-year students provided significant support for their second-year colleagues as they worked together in a team with the house officers. After the first terms each year the level of function of second-year students was so improved that it was difficult to distinguish between the second- and fourth-year students, a development which has continued to the present.

Three objectives currently shape the core clerkship in pediatrics: to understand the concepts underlying the discipline through work with patients in the hospital, nursery, and clinic and a series of correlated lectures; to acquire competence with the history, physical examination, and laboratory tests which are the basic tools of information gathering; and to appreciate the roles of all members of the child health team, including the nurse, social worker, recreational and physical therapists, nutritionist, speech and hearing pathologists, and others. Since September 1968, when Dr. Samuel Katz became Chairman of the Department, the ambulatory division of the Department has assumed new importance as a teaching site, with three and one-half full-time faculty assigned where previously there had been none. In this area each student is assigned patients for whom he has primary responsibility and to whom he then relates as a responsible physician surrogate. This realistic exposure to the primary care aspects of pediatrics is highly valued by a generation of medical students that has zealously sought primary care experiences. Emergency room and "walk-in" clinic experience is included in this rotation.

In addition to four weeks in the ambulatory division, each students spends three weeks on an inpatient rotation and one week in the full-term nursery. In each setting the student's function differs by virtue of the inherent characteristics of the area. A faculty tutor is responsible for each group of students on the inpatient rotation, but the student also works beside Pediatric residents, Family Medicine residents, and clinical faculty who are also practitioners in the community. Here the emphasis is on the teaching of the principles of general pediatrics. The physicians whose primary occupation is private practice offer weekly sessions, required of all students on the clerkship, which focus on such common pediatric problems as infant feeding, rashes, urinary tract infection, etc. During the week spent in the nursery the student devotes the major part of his time to examination of the normal newborn, with attention to those deviations which are clues to abnormal development and physiology.

Initially, much of the responsibility for day-to-day organization of the general clerkship lay upon the chief resident. With increasing experience it became apparent that more longitudinal direction and coordination of faculty and house staff required the designation of a specific faculty member for this role. Dr. Deborah W. Kredich, a member of the Ambulatory Division and a rheumatologist in the Department, has accepted these responsibilities. Students have been appreciative of faculty supervision of this phase of training.

A number of attempts have been made to evaluate the information which students acquire during their second year Pediatrics clerkship. Initially the department chairman and the chief resident jointly gave an oral quiz, twenty to thirty minutes in length, to each student. When this procedure started, the class size was eighty-six and there were approximately fifteen students per rotation. With increasing class size, there now are usually twenty-one students per rotation and the total time required for the individualized personal quizzes has become burdensome to schedule. For several years, therefore, the final examination was omitted. More recently, a written examination has been instituted at the end of the clerkship, and has been helpful in assessing some of the factual knowledge acquired by each student. At the end of each term the faculty and house staff meet to prepare a written evaluation of each student enrolled. Simultaneously, each student is asked to complete anonymously an evaluation of his clerkship experience. These evaluations suggest future modifications of the required course.

Fourth-year electives are custom-tailored to each of the subspecialty divisions and to the needs of such student constituencies as physicians associates, nurses, and psychology interns. For want of physical space, it has not been possible to continue a general pediatrics elective in the fourth year. During the seven-year period 1968–74, an average of thirty-three courses per year have enrolled students, with an average enrollment of less than two, which demonstrates the possibilities for individualized instruction characteristic of the elective curriculum. A summary of the enrollment of medical students in pediatrics courses is presented in Table XVII–1.

Table XVII–1. Numbers of medical students in pediatrics courses

Academic year	Fourth year[b] traditional curriculum	Second year[b] elective curriculum	Fourth year[a] elective curriculum
1966–67	82	–	–
1967–68	82	81	–
1968–69	82	87	–
1969–70	–	86	48
1970–71	–	86	58
1971–72	–	105	88
1972–73	–	105	56
1973–74	–	114	49
1974–75	–	114	49

a. Elective
b. Required

The fourth-year student becomes part of a team which includes faculty, fellow and resident. He sees patients in both the clinic and inpatient setting. As the term progresses, he begins to act, in concert with his teaching fellow, as a "consultant" in the particular discipline. These electives have been particularly helpful to students who are uncertain about career choice and wish to have further exposure to the field before selecting their postgraduate training focus. Additionally, they have been of help to students who wish to strengthen given areas of pediatrics, having already decided to embark on a child health career.

Each year approximately 18 percent of graduating medical students have elected postgraduate careers in some area of pediatrics. The majority enter pediatrics residencies directly; a minority spend an initial postgraduate year in general medicine programs before beginning advanced training in pediatrics. It is clear that, as these students move out from Duke, they value most the close personal and professional interchange among students, house officers and faculty which is encouraged by the elective system. They have, in nearly every instance, been among the outstanding members of the postgraduate programs they entered. While their initial success cannot with confidence be attributed solely to curricular change, it has been rewarding to observe.

XVIII. Psychiatry

Ewald W. Busse, M.D.

During the twelve years immediately preceding the inauguration of the elective curriculum, the Department of Psychiatry grew rapidly. There was a five- to sixfold expansion in the number of faculty members. The disciplines of psychiatry, psychology (including experimental, physiological, child, and clinical), sociology, and psychiatric social work were all substantially represented in the Department. This variety of specialties, plus a corresponding spectrum of research and clinical interests, made it absolutely necessary that the faculty members participate directly in curriculum policy and planning in order to guarantee effective teaching.

The clerkship

In planning the 1966 curriculum, the attempt to develop a "core" was largely motivated by the somewhat theoretical notion that in the core years it was important to learn the language of science, to learn to understand and appreciate the scientific method, to recognize that this information was applicable to the practice of medicine, and to achieve some knowledge in depth so that the student would have within himself a model for the type of learning and the extent of learning that would be required throughout his professional career.[1] In planning for the clerkship experience in the second year, therefore, it was not only necessary to respond to this theoretical challenge, but also to respond to the pragmatic approach of the skillful clinician. Our attempt to define a specific body of psychiatric knowledge and skill which is basic to all of the practice of medicine had then, and has now, two objectives: first, that the medical student acquire the skill and knowledge needed to recognize common and serious psychiatric disorders; second, that he gain some appreciation of the therapeutic approaches which are available to treat common psychiatric illnesses and be able to respond appropriately to serious problems until he can arrange for appropriate consultation.

As early as 1962 there had been discussions about the feasibility and the compatibility of the objectives proposed for the new curriculum. Some members of the Department felt that the objective of increasing the number of basic scientists, which presupposed a laboratory locus, and the goal of increasing the scientific orientation of physicians, which demanded a continuing clinical focus, could not be accomplished within one curriculum structure. It was proposed that the class be split in two, one part to follow the traditional curriculum and the other to follow the new course of study, in order, by comparison of the two groups, to test the assumptions on which the new curriculum is based. This proposal was rejected, however, for want of sufficient faculty, adequate facilities, and a selection process which would lead students to accept the division.

Since these early discussions, however, it has been the policy of the Department of Psychiatry systematically to survey the appropriateness of the content and the teaching effectiveness of the courses offered to medical students and to use the information gained to restructure our teaching efforts, not only from year to year, but throughout the academic year. It is the impression of the faculty that the social values and the attitudes of the student body do show significant changes, and that such changes affect their motivation as well as their expectation regarding the learning experience while on psychiatric rotation. Furthermore, the psychiatrists on this faculty include representatives of a variety of orientations, ranging from the biological approach to the psychoanalytic. To many students this has presented the opportunity for a range of exciting learning experiences. For others, who prefer the security of a single, hence relatively non-controversial, approach to clinical psychiatry, it has been anxiety-producing because of questions raised regarding therapeutic effectiveness, etiology, and diagnostic accuracy.

The structure of the elective curriculum, coupled with gradual increases in the size of the medical school class, forced the Department to attempt to devise a core curriculum that could be presented in a variety of clinical settings. Experience has proven that it can be accomplished, but only by the careful selection of faculty members who can respond to the particular clinical facility in which they are teaching and maximize its potentials as a teaching resource. For many faculty it is apparent that certain types of facilities are more readily and effectively utilized for teaching, for example, the medical-surgical services of a general hospital as contrasted to a mental hospital. This situation may not be as much dictated by the type of patient in the given clinical facility as by the system of care and the attitudes of the professional personnel involved in a particular medical or surgical unit. Attempting to teach psychiatry in a general or specialty clinic where the system is rigid and the personnel are uninformed, adversely affects psychiatric teaching efforts.

The clinical electives

The crucial period of work involving the development of clinical electives began in early April 1964. At that time it was decided to restructure the undergraduate curriculum committee of the Department of Psychiatry so that it would include two subcommittees. One of these subcommittees was to be assigned the responsibility of maintaining the current teaching effort, and the second was to devote its effort to the new curriculum. Dr. Fred Hine was chairman of the overall committee. On 4 April 1964, Dr. Hine presented to the entire Department a request for "a catalogue-style course description for each elective which will be offered under the new Medical School curriculum." By the fall of 1964, a tentative list of teaching areas which might be offered under the elective curriculum had been formulated. This tentative list was reworked and a number of new areas of teaching were added. The elective courses were not intended to provide a wide spectrum; emphasis was primarily upon offering electives by capable, interested faculty who had the facilities or resources to work with medical students.

At present more than thirty electives are offered by the Department. One-third of these are classified as basic science electives, the remainder as clinical courses. Some are offered in more than one term, so that the actual number of elective opportunities for the student in a given academic year exceeds ninety. Flexibility is increased, even within this broad range of choice, by allowing students to choose the course weight, and hence the level of concentration, in individual courses. Table XVIII–1 presents a summary of the elective enrollment experience of the Department. The most frequently chosen electives are the basic science courses in personality theory and development.

Table XVIII–1. Elective enrollment experience in the Department of Psychiatry, 1968–74

Year	Number of course sections	Enrollment: basic/clinical/total	Total units elected
1968	47	99/35/134	266
1969	52	89/60/149	289
1970	42	57/69/126	291
1971	33	31/39/70	146
1972	35	21/28/49	135
1973	43	60/44/104	214
1974	32	27/20/47	131

The clinical sophistication of students

During the first year of the new curriculum it was possible to compare the sophomores of the post-1966 curriculum with the juniors of the pre-1966 curriculum. After a few weeks of clinical experience, it was impossible to differentiate the sophomores from the junior students. Somewhat similarly our current impression is that the students during their first two clinical rotations suffer some loss in learning psychiatry while they are adjusting to the clinical setting; hence, these students during their first clinical exposure require more time from the faculty, and their learning experience is not as rewarding.

One continuing problem under the new format is how to make the distinction between clinical and basic science electives. Originally, the difference was largely determined by the identification of the type of department offering the course; that is, basic versus clinical. This gradually is changing so that the course content is the major determinant rather than the department offering the elective. The offering of electives by multidepartmental programmatic approaches has helped to improve clear presentation of content and teaching effectiveness.

Reference

1. E. W. Busse, "The Evolution and Impact of a New Medical Curriculum." *Seminars in Psychiatry* 2(1970):129–35.

XIX. Ophthalmology

Arthur C. Chandler, Jr., M.D.

The Department of Ophthalmology was established in 1965, one year prior to the introduction of the elective curriculum. Previously it had been a division of the Department of Surgery, and at the time of its formation as a department only one of the original faculty members from the division was still in the Department. The senior staff of Ophthalmology, then, had three members, who had attended Duke as medical undergraduates but who had received most of their post-graduate training elsewhere.

Under the traditional curriculum, Ophthalmology was allocated seven to ten days during the fourth-year surgical rotation. Each medical student attended a few conferences or lectures in a group and spent some time in the clinic. If an individual had no interest in the field, the time largely was wasted. If the student had a well-developed interest, frequently he could not be given enough attention because of the large number of patients being treated.

Under the elective curriculum, two lectures on ophthalmology are presented to each class as part of its introduction to clinical medicine. A second series of five lectures is offered during the second-year surgery rotation. Although necessarily abbreviated, this set whets the appetite of most students for additional exposure to ophthalmology. Since 1970, more than seventy students annually have elected to do additional work in the Department. A significant number of these select this work as part of their third-year program, both to be better prepared to return to the clinical services in the fourth year and to keep a bit of clinical "flavor" in the advanced basic science year.

Seven ophthalmology elective courses originally were established with varying ratios of basic science and clinical content and course weight ranging from one to eight units. A one-unit course entitled "Medical Ophthalmology," which includes one hour of didactic lecture and one hour of patient examination weekly, has been the most popular. In the longer courses, students are under the guidance of faculty members, and at advanced levels participate fully in the residency program except for assuming final patient responsibility.

Members of the Department agree that the student arriving on the wards at the beginning of his second year does not have quite the confidence of the third-year student under the traditional curriculum. He knows as much, but has not had as much time to develop facility in physical diagnosis and similar preclinical disciplines. But he rapidly catches up as the core clinical year progresses and, toward the middle of the year, no noticable differences appear between his capabilities and those of third-year students under the pre-1966 curriculum. Now, however, he still has two full years before him, with elective freedom in each. Gaps in scientific knowledge as it relates to clinical problems can be quickly closed.

In Ophthalmology, given a relatively small clinical staff and an unwillingness to have too much responsibility for student teaching fall on the resident physicians, the number of students choosing departmental electives has forced us to place limits on the size of courses and to ask some students to take a course earlier or later than anticipated. Apart from this minor logistical problem, the benefits of the elective curriculum to the department have been major. First, there is unquestionably a closer relationship between the staffs of the smaller departments and divisions, both medical and surgical, and the students. This is demonstrated not only by the number and variety of courses they elect, but also by the freedom with which unofficial advice is sought. Second, between 2 and 5 percent of each class that has graduated under the elective curriculum has elected ophthalmology as a career field, although nowhere near that number expressed interest in such a career as freshmen. Many of these students have compiled outstanding records in the better residency programs nationwide. We believe that this increase in the number of students opting for ophthalmology is attributable primarily to the success of the elective curriculum in providing a meaningful opportunity for early career decisions. The opportunity for elective research in the third year, correlated with clinical exposure in the fourth, strengthens their confidence in their chosen clinical roles by focusing directly on their personal interests and aspirations.

Special Study Programs and
Combined Degree Programs

XX. Medical Research Training Program

Nicholas M. Kredich, M.D.

The Medical Research Training Program (MRTP) was an early and clear declaration of the philosophy and intentions that shaped the new Duke curriculum. The decade of the 1950's witnessed the emergence in America of a strong national sentiment supporting efforts to eradicate disease. In response, the federal government initiated and sustained a well-financed system of support for biomedical research which was at that time the envy of the world and is now the envy of other researchers in this country. Medical educators projected creation of the equivalent of fifteen to twenty new medical schools by the late 1960's and anticipated the need to staff them with well-trained physician-investigators. It was in response to this anticipated need, and the influx into medical schools of bright, enthusiastic students motivated toward careers in investigative medicine, that the Medical Research Training Program was conceived.

Medical pedagogy at the time offered limited opportunities for the training of physician-scientists. One traditional pattern provided opportunity for an individual to enter a Ph.D. program immediately following medical school or after house staff training. The time commitments and financial requirements of these schedules, however, attracted too few students to satisfy anticipated national needs. More frequently, a young physician entered a research laboratory for one or two years of in-service training following his second year of medical school or immediately after internship and residency. The results of these experiences often were spotty, however, owing to students' lacking firm grounding in basic principles of research and to problems inherent in attempting training in busy research laboratories.

In 1958, under the leadership of Dr. Phil Handler and Dr. Eugene Stead, then Chairmen of the Departments of Biochemistry and of Medicine respectively, Duke responded to this set of problems with the introduction of the Medical Research Training Program. Its purpose was to provide selected medical students and house staff with an intensive nine-month experience in biomedical research in a setting free from other academic pressures and with minimum disruption of individual career plans.

The program focused upon the general topic of cell biology. Considerable deliberation went into the choice of this general training theme. Medical research prior to the 1950's had traditionally dealt with organ and whole animal systems, and consisted largely of descriptive phenomenology. While such endeavors had already proven (and continue to be) of considerable theoretical and practical importance, exciting progress in the fields of biochemistry, microbiology, genetics, cytologic ultrastructure and the then emerging area of molecular biology promised to unfold the chemical workings of the cell itself in a manner which would revolutionize the style of biological and medically relevant research. The content of our current curriculum clearly reflects the significance to medicine of the progress anticipated in 1958. The founders of the MRTP cannot lay unique claim to a special prescience by their recognition of the future significance of cell biology, but they certainly led the way in introducing these research disciplines to medical students in an innovative and effective manner.

Medical students entered the program at the beginning of their third year and, by taking clinical courses during the summers immediately preceding and following their enrollment in the MRTP and gaining credit for a senior elective term, could graduate on schedule with their classmates. Basic to the experimental nature of the program was the attempt to integrate the basic science instruction traditionally given in the first two years of medical school through additional training in the execution and interpretation of biomedical research. By combining this experience with the clinical training which followed medical school, Duke hoped to create a more effective and attractive continuum for training physician-researchers than previously had been available. It was expected that doctors at the house staff level also would profit more from this structure than from the "on-the-spot" approach to laboratory training. Duke house officers often were expected to take the MRTP as part of those subspecialty training programs largely focused upon research.

The program was well financed from the beginning, with starter grants from the John and Mary R. Markle Foundation, the Health Research Facilities Council of the National Institutes of Health, the Commonwealth Fund and the Trustees of Duke University. A new wing was added to the W. B. Bell Medical Research Building, which provided student laboratories, a lecture hall for the program, and research laboratories for several of the program's faculty. The Commonwealth Fund underwrote $75,000 in new faculty salaries for the first three years, and a large training grant from the National Institutes of Health provided funds for student stipends, laboratory equipment and supplies, guest lecturers and additional faculty salary support.

The spatial arrangements, conducive to close interactions among students and faculty, were important to the early success of the program, with faculty offices and program laboratories close together and adjacent to most of the research laboratories of the Departments of Biochemistry, Bacteriology, Physiology, and Anatomy. The equipment for the student laboratories included an electron microscope, walk-in cold and warm rooms, autoclaves, centrifuges, incubators, radioisotope counting equipment, spectrophotometers, facilities for microbiological studies, tissue culture facilities, and other items which made the student labs more modern and better equipped than most other research laboratories in the University. Even more important to the success of the program, however, were the four new faculty members recruited specifically for the MRTP: Dr. James B. Wyngaarden in medicine and biochemistry, Dr. Samson R. Gross in microbiology, Dr. Montrose Moses in anatomy, and Dr. Kenneth McCarty in biochemistry. Joined by Drs. William Byrne and Salih Wakil, who were already members of the Department of Biochemistry, they composed a faculty whose sole teaching responsibility was in the MRTP.

The course of instruction began with a sixteen-week block of time devoted to lectures and seminars in metabolism, enzymology, biochemical control mechanisms, microbial and biochemical genetics, cytology and ultrastructure, membrane transport, embryology, cell physiology and mammalian tissue culture. A large portion of this time was devoted to teaching basic laboratory skills through carefully selected experiments designed not only to reinforce classroom learning, but also to prepare students for the undertaking of their own research. Following this relatively formal and structured portion of the program, each student spent the next twenty weeks working on a small original research program of his own choosing and design. A preceptor was chosen from either the program faculty itself or from any other laboratory in the University engaging in basic biological research. By this time students were familiar with the special interests and knowledge of each faculty member, and were able to avail themselves of their advice whenever problems arose which were beyond the expertise of their own preceptors. Ongoing courses in mathematics, statistics, and electronics, as well as weekly seminars on topics of current research interest and on the students' own research projects helped lend cohesion to the program, even when the students had dispersed into many different laboratories.

Following the completion of the second year of the MRTP in 1961, Drs. Handler and Wyngaarden recorded their initial impressions of the program in *The Journal of Medical Education*.[1] They noted that the reactions and performances of medical students covered a broad spectrum ranging from unsatisfactory to outstanding. Of the eighteen students enrolled during the first two years, about half planned to pursue further their research training while the remainder intended to enter private practice. Many of the medical students were ambivalent about postponing their clinical training for an additional nine months, and were anxious about classmates' surpassing them in the acquisition of clinical skills. It is interesting to note the student suggestion at the time, that the MRTP might better follow six months of clinical experience. While the format of the new curriculum is designed to remedy the predicament experienced by the MRTP students many years ago, a certain amount of anxiety and ambivalence still is voiced by those who opt for a majority of clinically oriented third-year electives.

Handler and Wyngaarden described the post-doctoral students as more mature and in better perspective of their overall careers as possible physicians and scientists. For these individuals the MRTP was judged to be an unqualified success, an impression which continued to hold throughout the history of the program. Similarly, several faculty members from Duke and other universities found the program to be an excellent opportunity to refurbish their research skills and continue their educations.

A later evaluation of the MRTP was made in 1970 based on returns from questionnaires addressed to graduates of the preceding ten years. By that time 115 students had finished the program, about half as medical students and half as post-doctoral fellows. Of these sixty-five (57 percent) had completed their training and held positions with significant research and teaching responsibilities. An additional twenty-five students (22 percent) were still in training, but strongly indicated their intentions to pursue careers in research, giving a total of at least ninety students (78 percent) whose careers certainly profited by their experiences in the MRTP.

The sixteenth and final class graduated from the program in 1975, the program ending for reasons which can be enumerated but not easily quantified. The new curriculum, with its many tracks (more or less modelled on the MRTP), together with the development of the Medical Scientist Training Program from 1967 on, attracted some research-oriented students who otherwise might have entered the MRTP. Separation of the MRTP space in Bell Building from the new basic science facilities, opened in 1968, resulted in loss of the contact between students and faculty which was a unique aspect of the early years of the program. Termination of outside funding after the first years necessitated the assumption of new teaching responsibilities by the program faculty, most of whom now were involved in organizing and staffing the programs of the new curriculum. Finally, the increased social awareness and concern with the problems of health care delivery on the part of medical students everywhere in recent years has been accompanied by a general disenchantment with the accomplishments and potential of science for improving the quality of life for our citizens. As a result, a career as a physician-scientist probably appeals to a smaller percentage of students today than it did a decade ago.

The Medical Research Training Program was a successful educational experiment, judged either by the benefits it provided to students or by its capacity for suggesting new and larger designs. Its format served as the basis for many of the third-year specialty tracks of the elective curriculum, while a portion of its philosophy was adopted as the basic rationale for the curriculum overall. This assimilation assures that the influence of the MRTP will be felt at Duke for years to come until, inevitably, new approaches to medical education again supplant the old.

Reference

1. P. Handler and J. B. Wyngaarden, "The Bio-Medical Research Training Program of Duke University." *J. Med. Educ.* 36 (1961): 1587–94.

XXI. Medical Scientist Training Program

Thomas D. Kinney, M.D.

D. C. Tosteson, M.D.

Introduction

As plans for the elective curriculum neared completion in late 1964, planning was begun for a program that would provide an opportunity for highly qualified students who were strongly motivated toward careers in teaching and research in the medical sciences to obtain both the M.D. and the Ph.D. degrees. The primary impetus for this program was the need for well-trained faculty in the new and expanding medical schools throughout the country. That the Duke faculty had always been sensitive to this need is indicated by the Association of American Medical Colleges data showing that Duke ranked among the first ten medical schools in the country in terms both of overall research emphasis and percentage of graduates holding appointments on medical faculties.

Another stimulus was the recognition by the Duke faculty of the changing pattern of medical teaching since the end of World War II. Clinical teaching is now more often assigned to full-time scientist-clinicians whose scientific background and training enable them to teach the basic science material immediately applicable to clinical practice. Usually done at the bedside, such teaching is eagerly accepted by medical students because of its clear relevance to the patient and disease. The basic science faculty has greatly increased in number and is deeply involved in research. Its members are making discoveries that will be used by physicians of the future but may not yet be applicable to clinical practice. The subject matter they teach reflects the research interests of the basic science and their concern that students develop a scientific approach to the study of medicine. All too often, however, the basic science teacher, immersed in his own research interests, either forgets or does not have the background to relate the subject matter to the study of the patient, with the result that the basic sciences may be taught better than ever before, but without any discernible relevance to clinical medicine.

The Medical Scientist Training Program, in recognition of the special requirements for medical school teaching, was designed to prepare students for basic sciences careers shaped by significant clinical experience or clinical teaching careers broadly grounded in basic science principles and techniques. Whichever career orientation the M.D.-Ph.D. student chooses, he should be able to maintain a close correlation between scientific research and patient care, and hence become a more understanding and better medical school teacher.

Certain factors at Duke Medical School combined to make the faculty receptive to the idea of a Medical Scientist Training Program. First, there has always been a tradition of experimentation in the field of medical education since the founding of the school. Second, the basic science departments were also members of the Graduate School of Arts and Sciences and had extensive experience in graduate education in their respective disciplines. The faculties of all departments were willing to modify or change their educational arrangements if they could be convinced that an innovative plan could be devised. Most important, all the departments had a clear understanding of the educational needs of both graduate and medical students. At the time this program was under consideration, there were 150 graduate students enrolled in the basic science departments. In one sense, the development of a medical scientist program was recognition of Duke Medical School's extensive involvement in graduate education.

Another significant factor in the development of the Medical Scientist Program was the success of the Medical Research Training Program which is discussed elsewhere in this book. The faculty responsible for the program was successfully training selected third-year students in the principles and techniques of laboratory research to the extent possible within the time constraints of the undergraduate medical curriculum. The faculty which conducted this program was derived from all of the pre-clinical departments. Their experience was extremely valuable in planning the Medical Scientist Program.

Selection and support of students

All applicants to the Duke University School of Medicine receive a brochure describing the Medical Scientist Training Program with their regular application for admission. Upon admission to the School of Medicine, they may apply to the Medical Scientist Advisory Committee, which in screening applications looks beyond overall academic excellence for evidence of commitment to research, either in college or during summer employment, and for strong preparation in science and higher mathematics. The applicant pool is reduced to twenty, and each of these students is invited to Duke for two days to be interviewed and to become familiar with the school. Candidates then are ranked by the committee, and award notices sent in that order. A summary of this experience is presented in Table XXI–1. For 1976, the applicants offered positions or placed high on the alternate list have all, or nearly all, of the following credentials: grade point averages of 3.7 or better, MCAT scores of 95th percentile or higher in Science and Quantitative, research experience of high quality, enthusiastic recommendations, and high percentile rankings in the MCAT Verbal and General Information sections. These clearly are students with high potential.

The Medical Scientist Training Program has been supported from its inception by funds from the Department of Health, Education and Welfare, Public Health Service. The level of support has risen from almost $200,000 in 1966 to more than $500,000 for 1976–77. Most of these funds are used for direct student support. Stipends, beyond tuition and fees, currently amount to $3,000 annually for the first-year student and $7,000 for an advanced student whose attainments and experience are comparable to those of someone holding a doctorate. In addition, these funds help to support the more than thirty faculty members who regularly participate in the program and the large number of guest specialists who, by teaching in the areas of their special interest, provide a range of learning opportunities as wide as the range of student interest.

It was recognized from the start that this program would require a large input of faculty time. For this reason the staff was enlarged by six basic scientists and by six clinicians, all at the rank of Associate Professor. Although some new faculty were recruited from other schools, most positions were filled by Duke faculty who volunteered for the program. New faculty members were then recruited to assume the duties relinquished by volunteers. This nucleus of experienced faculty with primary responsibility to the program was enthusiastic and dedicated to the success of the program, and in time developed an esprit de corps which enhanced cooperation and communication. Other faculty members participated willingly for they found the students stimulating to teach. Soon they engaged in friendly competition to recruit these students into their research laboratories for work on their dissertations.

The combined degree programs: the core years

The first objective of the Medical Scientist Training Program is to provide each student with broad exposure to the major components of medicine and the medical sciences. In the first year, designated the core basic science year, the medical scientist student is exposed to a core of information from each of the preclinical disciplines as well as an introduction to the behavioral sciences, physical diagnosis and clinical microscopy. The faculty of each department presents those principles considered to be of greatest importance together with sufficient detail to document them. One great advantage of this introduction to the core material in each of the basic sciences is that it provides the prospective medical scientist with an opportunity to become acquainted with each before he is required to make a decision regarding his field of graduate study.

A multipurpose laboratory was designed for the students in this program. Construction was started only after an extensive study was made of multipurpose laboratories in other medical schools throughout the country. As a result, we have an extremely sensible laboratory incorporating the best design features of the laboratories that we visited. One area serves as a "home base" for the students during their first year. It has low benches which are comfortable for study and work with a microscope. Here the seating can be quickly rearranged for small seminars. There is a high bench area which can be arranged to provide any combination of benchwork needed for laboratory experiments or research projects. A separate laboratory contains equipment necessary for the preparation of the experiments as well as refrigerators, incubators, centrifuges, etc.

The laboratories contribute greatly to the operation of this program for they provide the setting and resources for much of the special instruction given to medical scientist students. Conferences and seminars are arranged for this group which provide greater variety of subject matter presented in considerable depth. Special laboratory exercises are devised for these students either because they have expressed a desire for additional information and study in a particular area or because their scientific background permits more advanced work.

These laboratories are unquestionably successful. They help develop a sense of unity and purpose in the group and provide a setting for the students to communicate freely and teach one another. They are suitable for the purposes for which they were designed and are highly regarded by the students. In fact, these laboratories served as a model for all of Duke's multipurpose laboratories when the school renovated its first-year teaching laboratories a year later.

Originally, we thought that the summer following the first year should be used either to allow the student to enroll in additional background courses in mathematics, chemistry or other fundamental sciences, or to begin graduate work or research. Experience has shown that most students either do not need additional background work or can acquire it during the school year, once they enter graduate school. We also found that the time available during the summer, because of vacations, was not long enough for any meaningful research to be completed. For these reasons medical scientist students are now advised to begin the core clinical science year immediately following the conclusion of the first year. This arrangement has the advantage of permitting them to begin their graduate school training in the spring of the their second year.

A comprehensive approach in medicine, oriented to the patient as a whole, is the basis for the second-year curriculum for the medical scientist. During this year, which represents the student's first introduction to clinical medicine, the focus is upon the total human biologic unit rather than upon separate organ systems. The experience is aimed at providing the student with the basic tools used in the practice of medicine. Each study synthesizes the material learned during the first year and applies it to the study of his own patients. During this year no attempt is made to cover systematically the entire body of clinical knowledge; rather, the student is provided a series of representative learning experiences based on the case study method. Our goals are to teach a method of approach to the patient, and to provide a firm foundation for the solution of new medical problems as they are encountered in the months and years ahead. It is our conviction that a solid year of experience in the major areas of the hospital, as participants in patient care and not merely as amphitheater spectators, will flavor the choices of research training by the students in a way that will relate their scientific efforts to the urgent problems of the sick.

The second-year curriculum is multi-disciplinary and interdepartmental. Stress is placed upon the continuity of biological processes–from conception through birth, development and maturation to senescence and death. Special consideration is given to the pattern of this developmental sequence in the individual, and to the changes in the pattern determined by genetic composition and by alterations brought about through the action of the particular environment in which the patient lives.

As it has developed, the year is organized into two periods. The first period, lasting for fourteen weeks, is devoted to Obstetrics and Gynecology and to Pediatrics; the second period, of twenty-one weeks, is shared by Medicine, Psychiatry and Surgery.

The first six weeks are spent on Obstetrics and Gynecology with considerations of the adult woman, sterility and infertility, conception, maternity and birth. Two weeks are then devoted to a combined interdisciplinary effort between the Departments of Pediatrics and Obstetrics in the area of maternal-fetal interaction, birth and the perinatal period. The next six weeks are spent on Pediatrics with emphasis upon normal development and the aberrations caused by disease in the young.

Medicine, Surgery and Psychiatry cooperate during the last twenty-one weeks of the year. During this period, a "mixed" ward (Strudwick) is set up and operated jointly by the medical and surgical departments. Each of these services assigns both senior staff and house staff to this ward, enabling both staffs to work closely together in teaching. The arrangement has worked well not only for the students but also for the respective staff members, who comment that they enjoy and profit from this experience.

At the same time, this arrangement has provided the psychiatrists with an opportunity to consult with the students and staff on patients who have psychiatric problems associated with their illnesses. Experience has demonstrated, however, that the "mixed" ward does not provide a sufficient number or variety of patients with psychiatric problems to give the student enough experience in psychiatry. Each student, therefore, is assigned to a neighboring psychiatric ward for a period of seven weeks. During this time the student is encouraged to continue to visit the mixed ward, to make rounds, and to follow the course of patients he or she has worked up while serving there.

A special series of seminars is held each year for the second-year medical scientist students. Outstanding clinicians are invited to conduct these seminars and to visit informally with the students, perhaps over lunch or dinner. This format adds a more personal flavor to the intensive introductory clinical experience and often aids the student in attempts to effect a meaningful integration of clinical and scientific efforts throughout the remainder of the program. Students in subsequent graduate research training years are similarly encouraged to return for selected hospital activities, and are frequently in attendance at clinical conferences, at grand rounds of various departments, and at the Clinical-Pathological Conferences held weekly throughout the academic year.

The advanced science years

The Medical Scientist Advisory Committee expected that students would spread out among a number of departments for the major concentration of their graduate work. This has proved to be the case, with a majority of students choosing to base themselves in Biochemistry, Physiology, Microbiology, and Pathology. Smaller numbers have enrolled in Anatomy, Behavioral Science, Psychology and Mathematics. All departments impose similar sets of requirements, which include: (1) completion of the course work necessary for the Doctor of Philosophy degree, (2) adequate performance in the Preliminary Examination, (3) original research suitable for a dissertation, and (4) successful defense of the dissertation in a final examination. The curriculum of each student is worked out in consultation with the Director of Graduate Studies of the department in which the student chooses to work and with the approval of the Medical Scientist Training Committee and the Associate Director for Medical Education for the School of Medicine, and the Dean of the Graduate School.

Students are encouraged to select courses relevant to their own developing individual interests rather than according to a prescribed program which is applied to all students in a given discipline. It is our view that such range, flexibility, and freedom are the essence of graduate education. Thus, candidates for a Ph.D. in physiology may take substantial course work in many related disciplines. If the student is particularly interested, for example, in the molecular basis of fundamental physiological processes like contraction, excitation, etc., he or she may take special courses in biochemistry, microbiology, cell ultrastructure, thermodynamics and mechanics, while a student interested in the integrative functions of the nervous system might take special courses in neuroanatomy, psychology and statistical methods.

The original research and dissertation of each student is supervised by a Faculty Advisor chosen by the student in consultation with the Director of Graduate Studies in his department. It is not required that the Faculty Advisor be a member of the department in which the student will take his or her degree. A student in the Department of Physiology, for example, may have an advisor in the Department of Biochemistry, provided that the plan meets with the approval of all concerned. Such arrangements have operated very successfully at Duke and again express our conviction that graduate

Table XXI–1. Summary of student experience in the Medical Scientist Training Program, 1966–75

Year	Applied	Admitted	Entering from non-funded	Leaving Program				Requirements completed for M.D.–Ph.D.**	Number of students participating during year
				Research elsewhere	Medical school	Graduated	Other		
1966	152	6	0	0	0	0	0	0	6
1967	209	6	1	0	0	0	1*	0	12
1968	221	6	0	1	2	0	0	0	18
1969	223	6	3	0	1	0	0	0	25
1970	227	6	0	0	2	0	0	0	28
1971	215	6	1	0	1	4	0	4	33
1972	292	6	0	0	1	4	0	4	36
1973	304	9	1	0	0	8	0	8	42
1974	349	9	1	0	0	9	0	9	44
1975	308	9	1	1	0	–	–	–	–

*Deceased

** Of the 31 students who have graduated from funded plus non-funded positions of the MSTP, three now have faculty appointments. All others are interns, residents, (or their equivalent) at excellent institutions.

education at its best is "tailor made" to the needs of the student. The Faculty Advisor serves as chairman of the student's supervisory committee which must include at least three members of the faculty of the major department. This committee generally administers preliminary (before commencing original research) and final (after completion of thesis) examinations to the student. For students in the Medical Scientist Training Program, both the Ph.D. degree and the M.D. degrees are usually awarded at the completion of the final clinical year. It should be emphasized that the participant who has achieved the Ph.D. degree is well suited to a future career as a staff member of a basic science department in a medical school.

The curriculum for the final clinical year is based upon the fact that an increasing number of academic careers are available in the field of medicine. The student is assigned an advisor from the clinical department in which he is most interested. Together they construct a highly individualized training plan for that particular student, one that places its major emphasis on the chosen clinical area but requires work also in a second clinical field. This year gives those who graduate from the Medical Scientist Training Program further training in clinical medicine to complement the core clinical year, so that the trainee's total clinical experience approximates that given in the regular clinical years of medical school. We intend that the student's last year provide experience that will not be repeated later during internship. Ideally, the future surgeon should be exposed to fields other than surgery, since he will receive intensive training in surgery during his residency. Students often are tempted to concentrate immediately upon their areas of special interest, and it is partially to offset this tendency that students are required to arrange their final clinical years in consultation with faculty advisors.

Conclusion

The length of time required for completion of the M.D.-Ph.D. requirements, added to the residency period, means that most graduates of the Medical Scientist Training Program are still in the advanced stages of their clinical training. Already some graduates hold full-time faculty positions, and the uniformly high quality of the residency programs to which the others have been admitted suggests that they will attain positions of similar responsibility. When these results are added to the faculty's enjoyment in the teaching of these students, it must be concluded that the Medical Scientist Training Program is a success.

Some 334 students have applied for entrance into the program for the 1976–77 academic year. Up to now funding has been adequate to support only 9 new students annually, and we expect that to be the case again this year, although at present we are assured of support for only 6. These outstanding applicants represent a perishable resource essential to the future growth and improvement of American medical research and teaching, and we hope they will be given high priority as alternative claims upon federal funds are evaluated.

XXII. Special Interdisciplinary Study Programs

Donald B. Hackel, M.D.

The Class of 1970 was the first to experience the basic science third-year curriculum, during the academic year 1968–69. A total of 193 elective courses were offered for their choice in building curricula. The number and variety of courses met one of the expressed objectives of the elective system in that students were able to explore their personal intellectual preferences and capabilities according to their individual backgrounds and career goals.

It soon became apparent, however, that the construction of curricula made up of relatively short periods of time tended to produce patchwork patterns of subjects. Students not infrequently chose courses on the basis of what they felt they most needed to fill in gaps in the first-year core; that is, for their remedial value. This approach was officially discouraged by advisors as contrary to the tenet that the third-year electives should provide an experience in depth in at least one major basic science area, and unofficially discouraged on the ground that students would have the rest of their careers to fill in gaps as necessary.

As early as June 1968, the Curriculum Committee had begun discussion of possible solutions to this problem. The suggestion most enthusiastically received was the establishment of Interdisciplinary Study Programs, with the Research Training Program serving as model. The RTP facility was made up of individuals with appointments in various departments, including Biochemistry, Medicine, Physiology, Microbiology, and Genetics. There were three main components to the Program: (1) A course. This consisted of lectures and laboratory sessions for the first three months, intended to give essential common background in biochemistry, genetics, and statistics. (2) A research experience. The last nine months of the Program involved work on a research problem, with a faculty member selected by the student. This was usually a mutually profitable activity and involved the student in an intensive basic science problem-solving experience. (3) A weekly seminar. This began during the second part of the Program, and served to keep the students in contact with each other, despite the fact that they were now working in scattered laboratories. Each student was made responsible for one topic, and his report served as the basis for critical discussion.

A procedural mechanism for development of additional interdepartmental study programs was established which prescribes the following steps:

1. The initiative for identifying areas in which programs should be de-

veloped comes from either of two sources: (i) the third- and fourth-year Curriculum Committee, or (ii) any faculty member who should discuss his ideas with the chairman or vice chairman of the third- and fourth-year Curriculum Committee.

2. The Curriculum Committee, after favorable review, identifies a Program Chairman. All department chairmen are advised of programs approved and invited to indicate whether or not they wish to contribute to them. Every department wishing to teach in a program has a representative on the Planning Committee, selected by the Department Chairman in consultation with the departmental Director of Medical Studies.

The Planning Committee consists of a representative of all departments involved in teaching, plus (in the case of basic science programs) two representatives from the clinical science departments or (in the case of clinical science programs), two representatives from the basic science departments. After the Planning Committee has been provisionally established, each representative discusses the program with his department chairman.

The Planning Committee is likely to differ from the Program Faculty, although the chairman of the Planning Committee is the Program Director. The Planning Committee role is organizational; its duties terminate after the program has received final approval.

Subsequent modifications of approved programs are discussed with members of the original Planning Committee and with the department chairmen involved in the program or its modification.

3. The Planning Committee members prepare a detailed program description, which they present to the Curriculum Committee and finally to the Medical School Advisory Committee for approval.

These guidelines were followed in the establishment of the first five programs developed on the RTP model. The programs were initiated, planned, and approved between September 1968 and February 1969, and began to function in the fall of 1969. These first five programs included the following subjects: behavioral sciences, cardiovascular-respiratory system, endocrinology, environmental medicine, and neurological sciences. They incorporated the three main components of the RTP: formal lecture course, seminars, and laboratory experience, although in some instances a library project could be substituted for a laboratory experience. All of them were programmed for the entire basic science year (thirty-six weeks in duration) although some students were permitted to drop out after one term (nine weeks) or after one semester (eighteen weeks) with proportional credit being given. They were offered in addition to the regular elective courses, and thus did not compromise the freedom and flexibility of the original system.

Each of these programs permitted enrolled students to take a limited number of departmental electives if they so desired although, to maintain the emphasis upon an integrated, in-depth effort, this was done with caution. For example, a few students taking the Cardiovascular-Respiratory Program also took the course in Cardiovascular Pathology which met Friday mornings for four hours for one term. Despite the freedom that was retained by this arrangement, however, a majority of students have preferred to organize their own curricula outside the Special Program's framework.

The primary reason given by students for their hesitancy to commit themselves to Special Programs was the concern that one full-year program excessively restricted their freedom of choice. Accordingly, when three new programs were organized for introduction in 1971–72, they were designed as single semester experiences. The Development and Differentiation Program arranged its coursework so that students could drop it after two terms or continue for four by continuing to work with a preceptor. The new Virology Program ran only for the first semester; the Immunology Program ran for only the second semester. Students participating for only one semester retained a greater freedom to enroll in departmental electives.

Table XXII–1 presents a summary of enrollment in these Special Interdisciplinary Programs over the past six years. Since a school year consists of four terms of nine weeks each, one student taking a Program for the full thirty-six weeks is counted as four student terms. Table XXII–2 describes the teaching effort devoted to these Programs as a percentage of the total teaching effort of the basic science electives.

Available records do not permit calculation of enrollment and teaching effort on a common base. However, these tables suggest that the percentage of teaching time devoted to the Special Programs was significantly greater than the percentage of each class enrolled in the Programs. Since a relatively large faculty was associated with each Program, close association of faculty and students resulted and was one of the major elements in their success.

As a means of evaluating student response to the Programs, a questionnaire was circulated to the sixty-seven students who took all or part of a Program between 1970 and 1972. There were fifty-five responses; of these, only three students said they would not take the same Program if they had the choice to make again. One student indicated that he would not choose any Program, while two said they would have taken another Program. It is of interest that of seventeen students who did not participate in a Program, when polled by a student committee in 1972, all indicated that, given the choice again, they would follow the same route and build individual curricula from departmental electives. Thus, both groups were, on the whole, satisfied; this speaks in favor of not being restrictive and of permitting as wide a range of elective options as the resources of a school will permit. Students clearly vary in their methods of study and in how they derive pleasure and profit from curriculum structures.

Most students who participated in Programs noted that the most valuable part of their experience was the laboratory work. Since this was a one-to-one tutorial arrangement, student satisfaction varied with the quality of the tutor. The formal lecture series was rated less valuable in almost all of the Programs. Student responses to seminars varied; one area of agreement

Table XXII-1. Enrollment in special interdisciplinary study programs, 1969–70 to 1974–75, by number of terms of enrollment

Course	Year 1969–70	1970–71	1971–72	1972–73	1973–74	1974–75
Behavioral sciences	23	12	14	13	22	4
Cardiovascular-respiratory	10	39	21	29	28	48
Development and differentiation	n.o.	n.o.	18	4	0	4
Endocrinology	20	20	23	24	12	28
Environmental medicine	0	4	1	3	n.o.	n.o.
Immunology	n.o.	n.o.	8	6	6	20
Neurological sciences	20	20	30	12	14	22
Virology	n.o.	n.o.	4	4	4	2
Research training	7	10	31	20	0	8
Total enrollment: special interdisciplinary study programs	80	105	150	115	86	136
Total terms of enrollment: all Medical School courses	408	452	412	512	504	552
Enrollment in programs as a percent of total enrollment in all basic science electives	19.6%	23.2%	36.4%	22.5%	17.1%	24.6%

n.o. = not offered

Table XXII–2. Teaching effort[a] in special interdisciplinary study programs expressed as a percentage of total teaching effort in third-year basic science electives, 1969–70 to 1974–75

Course	1969–70	1970–71	1971–72	1972–73	1973–74	1974–75
Behavioral sciences	8	4	5	4	6	1
Cardiovascular-respiratory	3	13	7	10	8	13
Development and differentiation	n.o.	n.o.	6	1	0	1
Endocrinology	7	7	8	8	3	7
Environmental medicine	0	1	1	1	0	n.o.
Immunology	n.o.	n.o.	3	2	2	5
Neurological sciences	7	7	11	4	4	6
Virology	n.o.	n.o.	1	1	1	1
Research training	2	3	11	7	0	2
Percent of total teaching effort devoted to special study Programs[b]	27%	35%	53%	38%	24%	36%

n.o. = not offered

a. Teaching effort is defined as the product of the number of students taking a course times the credit hours assigned to that course. Total Teaching Effort is defined as the sum of effort devoted to all basic science electives in a given year.

b. Percent of Teaching Effort is the ratio of effort devoted to Interdisciplinary Study Programs divided by Total Teaching Effort. (No allowance is made for students taking Special Programs who also took departmental electives.)

emerged in the suggestion that individual seminar sessions were most valuable to the student responsible for leading the discussion.

In summary, the special Interdisciplinary Study Programs have provided alternative pathways through the curriculum which continually have attracted a significant minority of each medical school class. The availability of these Programs keeps before all students the major objective of the third year, namely, study in depth in one or more basic science fields. Their availability also increases the freedom and flexibility which are characteristic of the curriculum generally. A faculty responsive to the new ranges of interests which incoming students present, through the design and revision of future Programs, will offer approximately the balance of choice and structure that many students seek.

XXIII. Biomedical Engineering Program

Theo C. Pilkington, PH.D.

In July of 1965, Dr. Douglas M. Knight, President of Duke University, appointed a University Biomedical Engineering Planning Committee to plan for the development of interdisciplinary programs involving engineering, medicine, and biology. After an eighteen-month study, this committee agreed that a formal administrative unit should be established to provide focus and coordination and to encourage the healthy growth of biomedical engineering at Duke University. In March 1967 a Division of Biomedical Engineering was established, and in February 1970 the Division became a Department. The Department is supported financially by both the Schools of Engineering and of Medicine, but reports administratively to the School of Engineering. Its purpose and function straddle the interests and activities of both schools, and the Department constitutes the primary focus for programs between engineering and the biomedical area.

An undergraduate program in biomedical engineering was initiated in May of 1967, and the first class of biomedical engineering majors graduated in 1969. Formal M.S. and Ph.D. programs were initiated in February of 1969, and in September of 1973, the undergraduate program became the first four-year biomedical engineering program accredited by the Engineers' Council for Professional Development. Undergraduates from this program have gone on to a wide variety of professional schools (medicine, mechanical engineering, zoology). The approximately 30 percent of the graduates who have not gone immediately into further training have been employed in industry and government in many occupations.

By allowing a continuity between medical school and graduate school, the new medical school curriculum of Duke University is particularly advantageous to students wishing to train for medical research by acquiring an M.D. and a Ph.D. degree. Students in this program must meet the requirements for admission as specified by both the School of Medicine and the Graduate School of Duke University. The first two years of the M.D./Ph.D. program in biomedical engineering are equivalent to the first two years of Duke's medical school program; in the first year the student is involved in basic sciences, the second year in clinical sciences. The following three years are devoted to obtaining the Ph.D. in the biomedical engineering program. During the first year of the Ph.D. program the emphasis is on graduate-level course work in engineering, math, and physiology, and in the latter years on research activities, but M.D./Ph.D. students are encouraged to begin early on a research program and there is no sharp demarcation between the period of course work and research. The "preliminary" examination which assesses the fitness of the candidate to carry out independent research generally marks the end of required course work and is generally administered some time after the first year and before the beginning of the third year. During the final year the student pursues clinical courses to complete the M.D. degree, thus acquiring both degrees in six years whereas normally this is a seven- or eight-year program.

A second advantage of this program is that it allows less "information-stagnation" than standard programs. By taking this integrated M.D./Ph.D. program one avoids the problem that occurs when the Ph.D. is taken first and followed by the M.D., in which case detailed knowledge of a limited field is forgotten or becomes obsolescent as new developments occur. Furthermore, the Ph.D. program, by intent, develops a pattern of questioning existing practices and precepts, while the M.D. program tends to stress best use of existing knowledge. Alternatively, if the M.D. is taken first, mathematical skills such as computer programming, differential equations, vector calculus, etc., which are little used in medical education become rusty, and considerable time is spent redeveloping previously acquired competencies. We have experienced some limited "information-stagnation" with M.D./Ph.D. students in the third year of the program who have not taken quantitative courses in the two years in medical school. A requisite to our Ph.D. course work is the ability to formulate physical problems in mathematical form and to work to solutions, and the M.D./Ph.D. students have reacquired this ability before the middle of their third year.

The first two years of medical school provide the prospective graduate student with an introduction to a variety of problems requiring solution, allowing him to choose his thesis topic prior to matriculation into the biomedical engineering program. Due to his proximity to clinicians, he is in a position to assess the appropriateness of his projected research and can enlist the aid of these clinicians in his research project. Since increasingly in engineering education today there are too many solutions begging for problems (e.g., modern control theory and theoretical mechanics) this is a significant advantage.

Further advantage to this program is that when the student returns to medical school for his final year, he is more mature than when he left it after his second year. He has a trained eye and is able to see many applications for the biomedical engineering knowledge he has acquired. In addition, he is better able to select those clinical rotations which offer promising research and development opportunities. Thus, broadly trained but with particular development in biomedical engineering approaches to problems, he should contribute new insights into the solution of medical programs through his further research, whether during residency or later.

Our experience with the M.D./Ph.D. program in Biomedical Engineering suggests that students selected for this program should have a strong background in mathematical, physical, and engineering sciences. It is extremely difficult to compensate for inadequate mathematical preparation. With this exception, however, the major requisites for success are the usual criteria of native ability and interest.

One disadvantage that appears on the horizon for the M.D./Ph.D. in Biomedical Engineering is that some students will be asked to postpone further research work until after their residency. Since residencies are usually three to four years, it is our anticipation that the student may experience an "information-stagnation," potentially reducing his research abilities below an acceptable level. This may be more of a problem with M.D./Ph.D. programs such as biomedical engineering than with programs in microbiology or biochemistry which are more closely integrated with clinical departments and programs. However, the Biomedical Engineering faculty are encouraged by the interest of some Duke clinical departments (and clinical departments at a few other medical schools) in developing an integrated research program as a part of the residency. Thus, we are hopeful that there will be residency opportunities that provide both clinically meritorious training and continuing research opportunities.

It is our conviction that the quality and potential of these students strongly indicate that they can make significant contributions to biomedical problems, but careful planning of all their opportunities is essential for the optimum development of these truly outstanding people.

XXIV. M.D.–J.D. Training Program

Eric Pfeiffer, M.D.

Johnnie L. Gallemore, M.D.

A unique program of combined and integrated professional education in both medicine and law was inaugurated at Duke in 1968. The ferment of curricular change in medicine, unequalled since the years following the Flexner Report, stimulated the development of curricula featuring substantial time for elective work in the basic and clinical sciences.[1] Joint degree programs appeared in which students worked not only toward the M.D. but also toward the Ph.D. in a wide variety of biological and social sciences. The Duke University School of Medicine pioneered in these areas, with the early establishment of its Research Training Program, the establishment of its new curriculum in 1966, and the introduction of its Medical Scientist and Medical Historian Training Programs.

The Duke University Law School had a similar tradition. The journal *Law and Contemporary Problems*, published quarterly from Duke, had for a decade given attention to such medical-legal questions as the problems of the aged, of drug addiction, of legal questions posed by the development of new technologies, and of Medicare. The decade prior to 1968 saw the enactment of a veritable flood of legislation (mostly Federal) in such areas as therapeutic abortion,[2] the training and licensure of subprofessional medical personnel,[3] organ transplantation,[4] and the "right to treatment" of persons involuntarily hospitalized in mental hospitals.[5] With an increasing number of Americans expressing the belief that access to medical care is a right rather than a privilege,[6] the need for interprofessionals bridging the fields of medicine and law seemed obvious given the complexities involved in government regulation of medicine, delivery of health care, and the application of new techniques.

While there has been some increase in recent years in the amount of medical, and particularly psychiatric, teaching in law schools, and of legal teaching in medical schools, the Duke program represents the first known joint degree program in medicine and law to be instituted. The goal of the M.D.–J.D. Training Program is to provide a small number of qualified individuals with a basic education in both fields, enabling them to function beyond the traditional interface of law and medicine, i.e. personal injury and malpractice litigation, in the areas of public policy and scholarly research.

The program assumes that an increasing number of promising career opportunities will become available, in government and the universities, for its graduates. Applicants are cautioned at entrance, however, that the mere possession of joint degrees has not been an automatic key to success. A preliminary research report by Curran indicated that the experience of 208 individuals with joint degrees in law and medicine had on the whole been less than satisfactory in terms of utilization of their skills in both of their fields of training. Most practiced medicine in one form or another. However, most of these were persons who obtained their education in a second field years after entering their first profession.[7] The needs of society described above are assumed to outweigh, for purposes of curriculum and career development, the experience of these earlier jointly trained professionals.

Applications for admission to the M.D.–J.D. program were first accepted and evaluated with reference to the 1968–69 academic year, and were limited to candidates who had not yet begun any professional training or who were enrolled in the first two years of medical school at Duke. Usually not more than three students are accepted in any one year. Table XXIV–I presents a summary of experience with applications for the five year period 1970–74.

Table XXIV–1. M.D.–J.D. applicants to the School of Medicine entering academic years of 1970–74

Year	Formal applications	Withdrawn prior to decision	Accepted
1970	10	0	1
1971	15	1	1
1972	30	1	2
1973	43	2	1
1974	49	3	4

For entrance into the M.D.–J.D. Training Program students must be admitted first to the School of Medicine, then to the School of Law, and finally pass screening by a joint Law-Medicine Committee composed of faculty from the two schools. Those accepted for the program enter a six-year curriculum with a basic structure similar to other interdisciplinary joint degree programs at Duke, but with allocation of time, particularly in the summers, peculiar to the demands of the overlap of law and medicine, as shown in Figure XXIV–1.

During the first year of law school the student begins his preparation with courses in Civil Procedure, Constitutional Law, Contracts, Criminal Law, Criminal Procedure, Property, and Torts. During the next two years he selects courses which are of special application to his medical-legal interests. The student's final year is spent in clinical elective work in the medical

Figure XXIV–1. Curriculum outline for the Duke University M.D.–J.D. Program

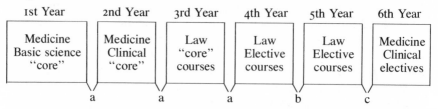

| 1st Year | 2nd Year | 3rd Year | 4th Year | 5th Year | 6th Year |

a. One quarter year of basic science electives must be completed in each of two of the first three summer terms; the third summer is not scheduled.

b. An optional summer medical-legal clerkship with a law firm is offered in the fourth summer.

c. Optional bar examination preparation may be scheduled for the fifth summer.

school. Balance is maintained in his medical education by the requirement of two summer terms of elective work in basic sciences. Throughout the six years the student has available the counsel of faculty members of both schools in the selection of courses and the definition of career objectives.

The rising number of increasingly competitive candidates for admission indicates the attractiveness of the M.D.–J.D. concept. Of more than 160 applicants during the year 1968–74, 7 withdrew prior to a decision on their applications and, of the remainder, 12 candidates were accepted. Of these, 4 withdrew prior to actual enrollment. Four currently are enrolled in the first two years of their medical training. One completed his medical training at Duke with the intention of obtaining his J.D. at another school. One withdrew from law school to complete his medical training. One elected to switch from law school to another joint degree program in public policy sciences. One completed his degrees and, after a straight internship and a one-year residency in internal medicine, accepted a position with the U.S. Public Health Service.

On the basis of this experience, assessment of the M.D.–J.D. Training Program after seven years must remain guarded despite the optimism engendered by the rising rate of applications. The obviously expanding interest in the program, locally and nationally, is offset to some degree by the limited enrollment and high rate of attrition. The experimental nature of the program justifies continued limited enrollments and careful screening of candidates, and high attrition is characteristic of a lengthy and demanding curriculum. However, two specific problems must be addressed if the rate of attrition is to be reduced. First, the program has been hindered by a lack of specific funding for either students or faculty. The prolonged period of student financial dependency under this program leads to increased indebtedness and drains on outside resources. Failure to achieve funding for faculty for this specific program leads to the second major problem: that there is an inadequate integration of interests and resources in the program both at the student and faculty levels. The few courses in either the School of Medicine or the School of Law which directly address problems arising from the overlap of the two fields are designed primarily for students who do not have the dual interests. The small number of excellent faculty members whose professional interests lie in both disciplines provide role models only on a spontaneous and informal basis in the absence of either undergraduate or graduate courses specifically designed for the joint degree program. Solution of these two problems would help to eliminate a third; namely, that the small number of highly visible M.D.–J.D. candidates do not have adequate support from most peers who, with interest in only one field, advance in their profession of choice at a faster pace.

It will likely be years before the careers of more than a handful of graduates of the M.D.–J.D. Training Program have developed sufficiently for meaningful analysis. Nevertheless, the obstacles inherent in its design provide meaningful challenge and the flexible, limited program is consistent with its experimental origin. The future vitality of the program appears to depend upon the validity of the assumption of society's need for its graduates and the success of the schools in overcoming the specific problems just described.

References

1. A. Flexner, *Medical Education: A Comparative Study*. New York: The MacMillan Co., 1925. For subsequent developments see V. Lippard, *A Half-Century of American Medical Education: 1920–1970*. New York: Josiah Macy Jr. Foundation, 1974. For the importance of the new Duke curriculum see pp. 24–26.
2. E. B. Stason, "The Role of Law in Medical Progress." *Law and Contemporary Problems* 32 (Autumn, 1967): 563–96. See also P. B. Thurstone, "Therapeutic Abortion: The Experience of San Mateo County General Hospital and the State of California," *J.A.M.A.* 209 (1969), 229–31.
3. E. H. Forgotson and J. L. Cook, "Innovations and Experiments in Uses of Health Manpower—The Effect of Licensure Laws." *Law and Contemporary Problems* 32 (1969): 597–619.
4. D. L. Stickel, "Organ Transplantation in Medical and Legal Perspectives." *Law and Contemporary Problems* 32 (1969), 597–619. See also A. M. Sadler and B. L. Sadler, "Transplantation and the Law: the Need for Organized Sensitivity." *The Georgetown Law Journal* 57 (1968): 5–54.
5. S. M. Goodman, "Right to Treatment: the Responsibility of the Courts." *The Georgetown Law Journal* 57 (1969): 680–701.
6. D. S. Burris, "Introduction: A Symposium on the Right to Treatment." *The Georgetown Law Journal* 57 (1969): 673–75.
7. W. J. Curran, "Interprofessional Education in Law and the Health Sciences: An Initial Report." Research Report for the Commonwealth Fund, New York, April, 1969.

XXV. Medical Historian Training Program

Gert H. Brieger, M.D.

In spite of strong historical interests on the part of many of the early members of the Duke medical faculty, there was never at Duke the occasional and unofficial course in medical history for medical students which was so common elsewhere in the United States. Prior to 1966, when the Medical Historian Training Program was inaugurated, the single most important contribution to the study of the history of medicine at Duke was the bequest by Dr. Josiah Trent of his personal historical library. During the 1940's Dr. Trent, encouraged by Dr. John Fulton of Yale, began to collect the library resources necessary to the development of a sound teaching program in medical history. Such a program clearly was one of his long-range ambitions, and only his untimely death in 1948 prevented Dr. Trent from establishing it himself. His superb historical collection became the nucleus of a still larger working library able to support both training and research in the history of medicine. The presence of the Trent Collection, nationally recognized and constantly growing, helped to keep the teaching obligation in view.

In 1966 two members of the medical faculty, Dr. E. Croft Long, Associate Dean for Students, and Mr. G. S. T. Cavanaugh, Director of the Medical Center Library and Curator of the Trent Collection, together with two members of the History Department, Professors I. B. Holley, Jr. and Seymour Mauskopf, drafted the outlines of a program in the history of medicine. They proposed a joint M.D.–J.D. program, six years in duration, aimed at producing young scholars for the field. The intention of the program was to attract a small number of outstanding students with interests in both history and medicine who ordinarily would not consider combining them in a single career. The program was specifically constructed to provide professionally trained medical historians to meet the current shortages of teachers and research workers in American universities. Dr. Genevieve Miller, surveying the status of medical history in American and Canadian schools of medicine at the time the Duke program was getting underway, documented these shortages. While the extent of competent historiography and the number of graduate departments in the history of medicine had increased since Dr. Henry Sigerist's previous survey in 1939, Dr. Miller commented that "The impact and influence of historians are still slight. Relatively few students graduating from North American medical schools today have a positive attitude towards history. Antiquarianism and mediocre teaching have tended to retard medical history in American medical education, and most medical educators today are unaware of its positive values. Only by being relevant and excellently presented will the subject be accepted as an essential part of the training of physicians." [1]

Dr. Miller found that nine North American schools offered graduate degrees in the history of medicine. Duke, although its faculty position was as yet unfilled, was one of these. Ten other schools of medicine had full-time professors teaching courses in the history and philosophy of medicine, but did not offer graduate degrees. The number of schools that offered courses had declined since 1952 to a total of forty-eight. Since in only nineteen schools was a department or professorship built into the medical school administrative structure, Dr. Miller commented that "60 percent of the courses are given by faculty members whose major activity is not medical history and whose qualifications to teach the subject vary considerably." [2]

Besides the continuing stimulus of the Trent Collection, the interests of members of the medical faculty and history department, and the nationwide need for qualified medical historians, the other significant stimulus to the initiation of the Medical Historian Training Program was the generous support of the Josiah Macy Jr. Foundation. In 1965 its Board of Directors established a program of support for the history of medicine and the biological sciences to stimulate both the teaching of the history of medicine in medical schools and to encourage students to take up graduate study in the field. Another principal aim of the Foundation was to strengthen the relationships between medical schools and their parent universities.

All of these goals were realized by the program of fellowships awarded to students in the newly designed M.D. – Ph.D. program at Duke University. The Macy Foundation pledged to support a small number of students with full tuition plus stipends for the entire six years of their studies. The first student, Russel C. Maulitz, enrolled in 1967. An additional student began in each of the succeeding three years. In 1970 Dr. Gert H. Brieger joined the medical school and history department faculty to direct the program.

The students follow the same course of studies as their medical school classmates for the first two years of their studies. The third and fourth years have been devoted to graduate study in history. All students in the program have worked closely with Professor Seymour Mauskopf to set their study of medicine in the more general context of the history of science. Although each student is free to design a Ph.D. program according to his individual interests, a majority have chosen to extend this process one step further by concentrating some of their elective time in social and intellectual history, of which the history of science is a subset. Professor I. B. Holley, Jr. offers this opportunity to students particularly interested in American history, while Professor Harold Parker teaches a similar course focused upon European history. Dr. Brieger offers individual advanced tutorials in the history of medicine. The close relationship of the Medical Historian Training Program to the graduate studies offered by the History Department has given the history of medicine program a strength it could never have achieved on its own.

Of the final two years, the students generally have spent approximately one in medical school elective courses and one in writing their dissertations. All summers have been fully utilized as well, either in language study, preparation for the Ph.D. preliminary examination or for research.

Dr. Maulitz received his degrees in 1973. After two years of internal medicine training he joined the faculty of the University of Pennsylvania with a primary appointment in the Department of History and Sociology of Science and also in the Department of Medicine.

Dr. Robert C. Powell earned his degrees in 1974. After a year of psychiatry training he joined the History Department as well as the Medical School of the University of Missouri, Kansas City. He will, in subsequent four-month summer periods, finish his psychiatry residency.

Dr. Peter English graduated in 1975 and joined the pediatric house staff at New York Hospital. One of the original four Macy-supported students and two additional ones are still in various phases of their training.

The original objective of the Medical Historian Training Program, to provide trained medical historians for academic courses, seems to have been fulfilled thus far, although it is still too early to say with certainty what careers the graduates will pursue. In addition, the M.D.–Ph.D. program has stimulated an increased interest in the history of medicine among both undergraduates and medical students. Elective courses in the history of medicine, available in the medical school since 1970, have enrolled a small but steady number of students each term. The presence of the M.D.–Ph.D. students in the medical school classes also has raised the level of interest of fellow students in the history of medicine.

References

1. Genevieve Miller, "The Teaching of Medical History in the United States and Canada, Part I." *Bull. Hist. Med.* 43 (1969): 267.
2. Ibid., p. 263.

XXVI. M.D.–M.P.H. Training Program

E. Harvey Estes, M.D.

In 1964, the Department of Preventive Medicine was reorganized, as described in Chapter XII. As a part of the effort of this new department, Dr. E. Croft Long and Dr. William J. A. DeMaria designed a program to provide medical students with a unique series of experiences in community medicine through the combined facilities of the Duke University School of Medicine, the University of North Carolina School of Public Health in Chapel Hill, and the University of San Carlos School of Medicine in Guatemala. Under this proposal, students would receive their basic medical education at Duke. Arrangements were made for a series of lectures and seminars in epidemiology, biostatistics, socio-economics, social anthropology and related topics, principally at the University of North Carolina School of Public Health. Field experience in community medicine in Guatemala and Nicaragua was offered through the cooperation of the University of San Carlos. Limited funds for student support were obtained for this program in 1966 and, beginning in 1967, four Duke students participated.

This program led to interaction and cooperation between Duke, through Dr. Long, and the faculty of the University of North Carolina School of Public Health. Dr. Long, in these conversations, suggested that a joint M.D.–M.P.H. degree program, with the M.D. degree to be awarded by Duke and the M.P.H. by the University of North Carolina, might be established. The elective options of the new Duke curriculum and the patterns of cooperation already established with Chapel Hill and San Carlos would be the organizational basis for it.

The proposal for a joint M.D.–M.P.H. degree program was approved in 1967 by the medical faculty at Duke and the faculty of the University of North Carolina School of Public Health. The first two years of the program were the core basic science year and the core clinical science year of the new Duke curriculum. The student then transferred to the School of Public Health for the four academic semesters and one summer session required for the Master of Public Health degree, taking a sequence of courses in Epidemiology, Biostatistics, Public Health, Health Administration, Environmental Sciences and elective social science courses, besides conducting a field investigation leading to a thesis.

The original proposal specified that, upon completion of work for the M.P.H. degree, the student would return to the Duke University School of

Medicine for a final year devoted to clinical science electives selected to complement his previous experiences and particular career objectives. During discussion by the Duke Medical School Advisory Committee, however, the question was raised concerning the desirability of allowing students to bypass entirely the basic science electives normally available to third-year medical students. It was decided to allow six months of elective credit toward the M.D. degree for students who completed the M.P.H. curriculum. This elective credit was to be equally divided between basic science credit and clinical credit.

The decisions to credit students completing the M.P.H. degree with less than a full year of work toward the M.D. and to divide the six months credit equally between basic science and clinical experience reflect a fundamental problem encountered by this joint-degree program. Modifications of the medical curriculum toward the social sciences or other non-traditional content met with resistance from those who feel that the social sciences and, to a lesser degree, epidemiology and biostatistics, are less valid as a background for medical practice than the traditional basic sciences. This primarily explains the compromise that assigned credit be equally divided between the basic science and clinical areas, though the course content of the M.P.H. program is not directly related to the care of the patients. Given the assumption that the two core years of the Duke curriculum provide an adequate groundwork for medical practice, then an entire basic science year spent in Public Health should not do violence to preparation for a medical career. This is especially true since the focus of the public health curriculum is upon problem-solving.

A second major problem affecting this program has been lack of adequate funding for scholarship support. Without financial support, anticipated student demand for the program did not materialize immediately. One student was admitted to the program in 1971–72, two were admitted in 1972–73, and two more in 1973–74. The majority have elected a concentration of courses in health care planning. One student elected to pursue epidemiology as a "specialty," taking his work at the Harvard School of Public Health instead of the University of North Carolina School of Public Health. Currently, two graduates of the program are engaged in public health activities: one is director of a state health department and the other is working with the Agency for International Development in Central America.

In summary, the M.D.–M.P.H. Program, as it evolved out of a desire to provide interested students with an exposure to environments in which preventive medicine has an equal role with remedial medicine into an intensive course of studies, symbolized by the joint degrees, represents the type of flexibility in structure and opportunity which was a major goal of the new curriculum. In contrast to some of the other joint degree programs, it lacks outside support funds and consequently has been less well subscribed. Nevertheless, it has been utilized by a total of five students, two of whom already are using their training in an effective and productive manner in the field of public health. The increasing concern of Americans for improvements in the public health field gradually should overcome the problem of non-acceptance by those faculty members who view the course content as being less acceptable than traditional basic sciences as a background for medical practice.

Evaluation

XXVII. Educational Activities Analysis of the Elective Curriculum

Thomas D. Kinney, M.D.

Jane Elchlepp, M.D., PH.D.

William D. Bradford, M.D.

Introduction

The elective curriculum was designed specifically to give the student more freedom and flexibility than were available in the traditional curriculum. It enabled each student to utilize more fully the resources of the entire university, as well as those of the medical school, in shaping medical studies to fit chosen career fields. In a sense, this was a modification of the undergraduate university system in which basic or introductory courses are followed by a wide range of elective courses. The elective courses, therefore, became the keystone of the medical school curriculum, and success or failure of the curriculum became dependent upon their quality and organization.

In developing the electives, the stated goals were: first, to acquaint the student with a variety of disciplines from which he could make a career choice; second, to stimulate study in considerable depth in an area of particular appeal. The faculty was urged to design electives that would demand rigorous scholarly effort, whether through coursework, laboratory experience, a research problem or a clerkship. To faculty members who were interested in teaching, electives were seen as challenging, for they gave the teacher great freedom to present ideas and to share scientific and clinical experience with students. The following pages assess the effect of this challenge in terms of institutional growth, transfer of information, patterns of elective choice, expenditure of teaching effort and success as measured by national norms in sustaining levels of educational achievement.

The dynamic setting of the curriculum

The decade of the 1950's was a period of national concern about the status of science in America. There was emphasis upon and a remarkable growth in research and the production of research manpower. By the mid-1960's, national concern had shifted to the availability and production of manpower for medical care. By 1970, when the first class under the elective curriculum was graduated, the pressures for increasing physician manpower were great and had been expressed in such projects as the physician augmentation program. More recently, quantitative concerns about medical manpower have been gradually replaced by increased attention to the character of health care delivery systems and to utilization of medical and allied medical manpower. Thus, it could be said that *planning* for the new curriculum occurred during a period of intense emphasis upon biomedical research, that *implementation* of the new curriculum occurred during a period of emphasis upon medical manpower production, and that modification of the curriculum for subsequent classes of students was conditioned by concern about health care delivery systems and the quality of health care itself.

The internal institutional environment has been as dynamic as the external environment. Between 1960 and 1966, the planning years, eight new department chairmen were named. By 1970, four additional chairmanships had changed hands and two new departments had been created. In 1961, a long-range planning report called for increased development of research resources and improvement of the basic science departments. These recommendations, coupled with the resource requirements of the new curriculum, produced a considerable expansion in both faculty and facilities.

These internal changes combined with the nationwide emphasis upon increasing medical manpower resulted in increases in admissions in 1967, 1970, and 1972. Six student generations have experienced the elective curriculum (classes of 1970–75), but between 11 percent and 15 percent of each of those classes took three to five years longer than usual to graduate because of participation in combined degree programs or other extended study provided in elective opportunities. The growth of the faculty and student body since 1966, presented in Figure XXVII–1 must be understood against this backdrop of change and flexibility.

Figure XXVII–2 examines this growth in terms of changes between the basic science and clinical science faculties and in terms of the variation in numbers of first- and third-year students (who draw primarily upon basic science department resources) and second- and fourth-year students (who draw primarily upon resources of the clinical departments). The variations which show up in the number of students in these two groups reflect both the changes in class size and the enrollment in combined degree programs. In 1968–69, for example, twelve students who would otherwise have been included in the basic science elective group transferred to the graduate school for combined degree programs. By 1972–73, this number had risen to forty-four. These students received third-year medical school credit for their graduate work and returned, on an irregular basis, for their fourth-year clinical electives. Such variations combined to make forecasting of load and resource requirements for the third and fourth years quite difficult.

Fortunately, overall institutional growth overcame these difficulties during the transition from one curriculum to the other. The development of three new departments, expansion of clinical bed facilities, additional affiliations with community and regional hospitals, establishment of a Comprehensive Cancer Center and new outreach patient care programs as well as a wide variety of other programs supported the steady increase in faculty necessary to the success of the new curriculum. Since each innovation influenced the environment, and hence the thinking of students and faculty alike, the curriculum experienced by the class of 1975 was quite different from that experienced by the class of 1970.

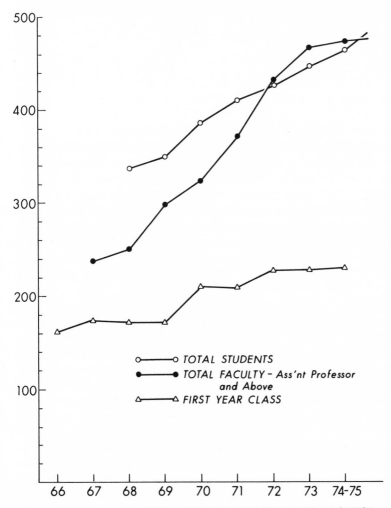

Figure XXVII–1. Growth in faculty and student body under the elective curriculum

The advisory system

The informal grapevine by which information about the Duke experience passes to students from other students and from faculty and staff has been mentioned frequently in previous chapters and, since similar processes operate in all medical schools, does not require further description. In more formal terms, students are encouraged in time of academic or personal distress to seek out any faculty member or administrator with confidence that the conversation will not become a matter of record. The student may also elect to have a faculty member from his or her department of major concentration act as a personal advisor on an ongoing basis. In each department, the chairman canvasses the faculty for volunteers to act in this capacity; each is matched with one or two students on the basis of common interests. The personal advisor commits himself to regular, informal meetings with his students, and usually does not accept formal advisees in successive classes. A little more than half of the students in each class select a personal advisor.

Each student also has a departmental professional advisor for all phases of

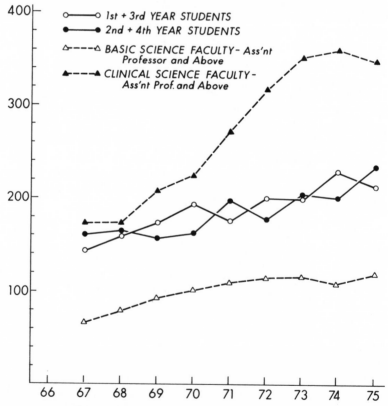

Figure XXVII–2. Growth in faculty and student body in the basic and clinical sciences

his or her medical career. As a practical matter, most of this advice is focused upon selection of courses in the elective years as preparation for postgraduate training and future careers. Six months before the second year, when students register for their first electives, an open meeting of the class is held. Procedures of the elective system are reviewed, a catalogue describing all basic science and clinical electives and special study programs is distributed, and each departmental professional advisor summarizes the offerings of his department. After his meeting, students choose a professional advisor in the basic science department and clinical department in which they intend to take the major portion of their elective work. The departmental professional advising role is the key to making the elective system work to the benefit of each student, for the advisors not only approve students for work in individual courses and departments but also certify, to and for each student, that the goals of the new curriculum are met in the elective choices made.

One month before registration for the third year, all rising third-year students appear before an advisory screening panel for a broad review of their educational aims and course selections. These panels are composed of one basic scientist, one clinical scientist, and a chairman who is usually a faculty member experienced with the curriculum and who may be either a basic or clinical scientist. The students are asked to describe their course selections in view of career direction and receive anticipatory guidance. While many students feel threatened by this procedure, the Screening Panels are advisory only and major disagreements on course selections revert to the professional advisor and Office of Undergraduate Medical Education for resolution.

The Screening Panel has two major virtues: first, the student is supported in the choice of courses by broad approval; and second, faculty are drawn into curriculum planning. Once panel approval is given to a student, modifications in course or career plans are made through the departmental professional advisors.

Since most rising seniors have a firm idea about their career direction and courses they may or may not wish to take, they do not appear before screening panels. Instead, rising seniors construct their courses of study with their professional advisors. In addition, they begin to plan their postgraduate education with the postgraduate program director in their area of major concentration.

At the beginning of the last academic year of undergraduate medical education, the senior student has an interview with the Associate or Assistant Director for Undergraduate Medical Education to provide information for the official letter of recommendation and other credentials necessary for obtaining a postgraduate position. After this interview the student is encouraged to consult the departmental chairmen and postgraduate program directors who can be expected to write personal, supporting, and usually determining letters on the student's behalf. In constructing the "Dean's Letter," the Director attempts to describe the student's outstanding talents, accomplishments, and extracurricular contributions in medical school and also in college. Since an increasing number of postgraduate training programs will not interview prospective house officers until the "Dean's Letter" is at hand, these letters are mailed early in the fall of the student's last academic year. Supplementary material which could enhance the student's application, such as election to Alpha Omega Alpha or honors grades, is provided in later mailings.

Monitoring the curriculum

The transfer of information through the advisory mechanism is the first stage in the process of monitoring the curriculum. Both faculty and students sit on the curriculum committees that review all of the academic activities in the School of Medicine. During the process of planning the elective curriculum, these committees were created to set the goals for and organize the material to be presented in each academic year. After 1966, the curriculum committees were continued to provide for stability, orderly change and evaluation.

Each of the four committees consists of two faculty members from each discipline participating in the current year's programs, and four students selected by the Davison Society, which constitutes the medical school student government. The Director of Medical Education, the Associate Director, and the Registrar serve ex officio on all four committees, each of which has the following areas of responsibility: (1) evaluation of content and quality of the year's courses; (2) attainment of a proper balance of subject matter, integration of that matter into the learning experience for the year, and elimination of repetitious subject matter; (3) scheduling for all major and minor courses avoiding time conflicts where possible; and (4) evaluation of teaching methods and the learning experience of the students.

So that the entire curriculum may be coordinated and flexible all four curriculum committees serve in an advisory capacity to the Medical Education Policy Advisory Committee (MEPAC), which coordinates and schedules all programs and courses in the medical school and sets policy for all educational operations short of major restructuring across departmental lines. This committee is chaired by the Director of Medical and Allied Health Education and composed of two basic science and two clinical science departmental chairmen, the chairman of each curriculum committee, and student representatives and appropriate administrative officers. It reviews all matters of educational policy and the activities of the four curriculum committees. MEPAC is finally responsible to the Medical School Advisory Committee (MEDSAC), the executive committee of the School of Medicine.

Each year, at the close of the spring term, a two-day conference on medical education is held at Quail Roost Conference Center in Bahama, N.C. All curriculum committees and appropriate administrators and students participate in these meetings. Traditionally, student and faculty critiques of course and curriculum material are presented and discussed. In addition, broad subjects such as admissions, residency training, advisory system and postgraduate education are formally reviewed. Major resolutions passed at the yearly Quail Roost Conference appear on subsequent MEPAC agendas and are assigned to the proper curriculum committee for review and implementation if feasible. The material which follows was considered, year by year, at these conferences.

Patterns of elective choice

The new curriculum projected the maintenance of a balance in the elective choices of the students, 50 percent in basic sciences and 50 percent in clinical sciences. As seen in Figure XXVII–3, third-year students have tended to cross over and pick up clinical science elective credit. Their preference for clinical electives undoubtedly reflects the student interest and commitment to a career in clinical practice. This was disappointing to members of the basic science departments, who had hoped that the students would return from their clinical experience to study related basic material with a new perspective and with renewed interest. Equally disappointing was the reluctance of students to avail themselves of science courses offered elsewhere in the university. Fortunately, the clinical chairmen were unanimously agreed upon the importance of basic science to the practice of all disciplines of modern medicine and they strongly supported the concept that the time spent in the elective years be divided equally between basic and clinical science. As time passed, the experience of the earlier classes with the basic science electives led to a better understanding of their value so that succeeding classes accepted the arrangement with less hesitation.

Within the basic science elective pattern, the number of students electing special study programs, as opposed to general basic science electives, varies greatly from year to year. Once again, the changing environment enters into review of the data. In 1968–69, only three special study programs were offered, and enrollment was correspondingly low. In 1971–72, there were nine, and enrollment rose to more than 50 percent of the total enrollment in electives, as measured by credit hours awarded. Since then, fluctuation has continued, probably reflecting the success of program designs in anticipating needs perceived by the students (see Figure XXVII–4).

Figure XXVII–5 shows the distribution of elective credit hours on a percentage basis, exclusive of special study programs, among the basic science departments. Analysis of specific course enrollments indicates a clear bias toward electives with clinical correlations. Since 1972–73, the majority of elective credit hours has been split among Pathology, Microbiology-Immunology, and Physiology-Pharmacology. Other departments show minor fluctuations and gradually decreasing percentages of total enrollment.

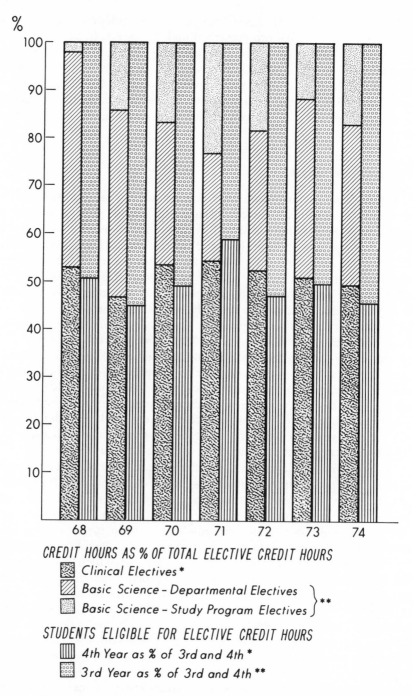

%

CREDIT HOURS AS % OF TOTAL ELECTIVE CREDIT HOURS
  Clinical Electives*
  Basic Science – Departmental Electives ⎫
  Basic Science – Study Program Electives ⎭ **

STUDENTS ELIGIBLE FOR ELECTIVE CREDIT HOURS
  4th Year as % of 3rd and 4th *
  3rd Year as % of 3rd and 4th **

Figure XXVII–3. Distribution of elective credit hours among third-and fourth-year students.

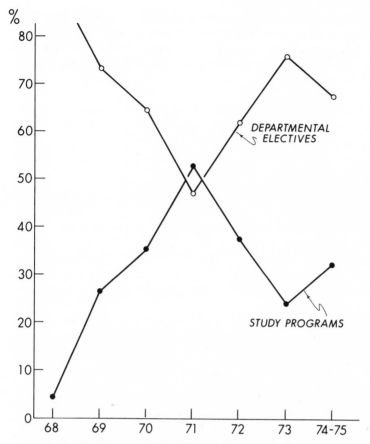

Figure XXVII–4. Patterns of enrollment in basic science (third-year) general electives and special study programs.

In Anatomy, the most consistent credit-hour enrollment has been in a course in surgical neuroanatomy. During the first two years, the most popular elective course in Biochemistry was "Biochemistry of Disease." During the last two years, a nutrition course has gained increasing popularity, although the principal enrollment in the Biochemistry Department continues to be in research courses. In Community Health Sciences, basic science enrollment has shifted away from courses relating to the use of computers in medicine to those analyzing health care systems. Microbiology, which since 1970–71 has expanded significantly as a department, particularly in the area of virology, has seen its heaviest enrollment in courses emphasizing diagnostic applications and the pathophysiology of infectious disease. In Pathology, enrollment is spread evenly across a variety of organ-system courses, with some preference indicated for courses in the pathological basis of clinical medicine, cardiovascular pathology, and autopsy pathology. Although the course offerings in Physiology-Pharmacology have changed frequently, the largest share of enrollment over the years has been in courses with the word "clinical" in their titles. In Human Behavior, no clear preference patterns emerge.

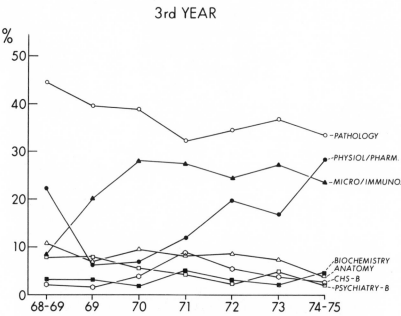

Figure XXVII–5. Distribution of elective credit hours in basic science courses, exclusive of special study programs

Figure XXVII–6 shows the distribution of elective credit enrollment among the clinical departments. In all departments, there is increasing student preference for clinical preceptorships involving patient care. The trend toward higher enrollment in Medicine, which has been primarily at the expense of enrollment in Surgery and Pediatrics, may reflect those two departments' practice of advising students to concentrate their electives outside their intended career fields in order to be more broadly prepared for specialized postgraduate training. This appears to be a direct result of the new curriculum's success in facilitating early career choices by the students.

During the years of the elective curriculum, the grade point averages of most students have tended to rise year by year (see Table XXVII–1. This rise has paralleled the improvement of the MCAT scores presented at admission. Because it also occurred during a period when average grades have risen in all types of institutions of higher learning, the contribution of the

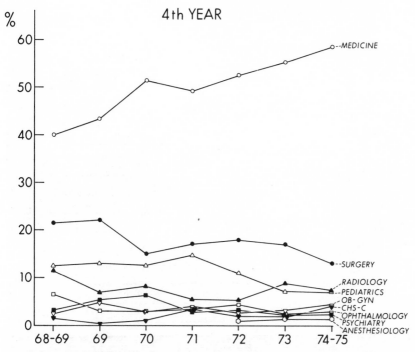

Figure XXVII–6. Distribution of elective credit hours in clinical science courses.

Table XXVII–1. Comparison of average MCAT scores and class quality point averages, classes entering 1964–74.

Enter year	M.D. year	Number of students enrolled	Number of M.D.'s*	Average MCAT	Class grade point average
1964	1968	82	84	595	2.9
1965	1969	82	76	579	2.8
1966	1970	81	70	601	2.9
1967	1971	87	80	618	2.9
1968	1972	86	98	614	3.1
1969	1973	87	91	631	3.3
1970	1974	105	97	609	3.4
1971	1975	105	105	599	3.5
1972	1976	114		612	3.6
1973	1977	114		633	3.6
1974	1978	115		618	3.6

*Includes some transfer students.

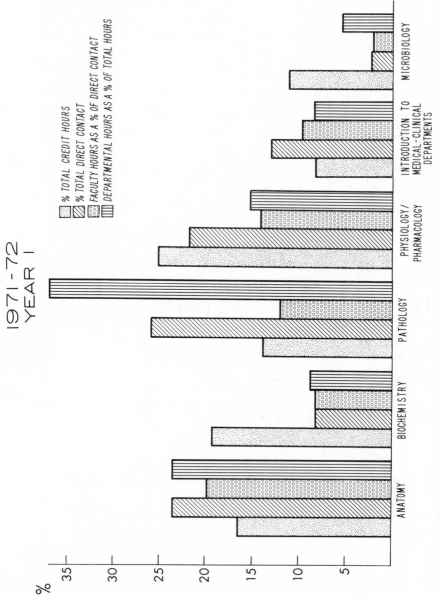

Figure XXVII-7. Comparative analysis of department effort in the first-year curriculum, 1971–72

change in curriculum structure to this improvement cannot be measured accurately, even though the faculty is satisfied that the grades earned by students in recent classes do reflect their performance.

Departmental effort analysis

During the academic years 1971–72 and 1972–73, data was collected to assist in the assessment of the undergraduate curriculum utilization of resources. The data was collected by a combination of questionnaires and interviews, in some cases including actual accompaniment of faculty or students by data collectors for up to four or five days. The data was organized by course around this basic question: "What do you need in the way of staff, space, time, and other resources in order to teach this course?"

In the data collection, resource utilization was identified according to the departmental origin of the specific resource. Thus, if a course offered by one department used personnel from other departments, their effort was credited to the department of origin rather than to the department responsible for the course. It was felt that this would be of value in identifying departmental loads that were not being credited to those departments by the assessment of credit hours.

The data was difficult to interpret in terms of cause and effect. At first glance, there seemed to be a marked increase in faculty and faculty time required for teaching. Closer examination showed that this was not entirely true since the increase in numbers of both basic and clinical faculty could be correlated with the development of research and clinical care programs not primarily related to teaching medical students.

Clear objective data on teaching and support utilization could be obtained for the first curriculum year. In the second and fourth clinical years, it was difficult to allocate the "joint product" effort of faculty engaged simultaneously in patient care, research, undergraduate teaching and postgraduate teaching. A similar problem arose with the analysis of the third-year teaching; it was difficult to separate research activity and the concurrent teaching done for the individual student.

Figure XXVII–7 compares credit-hour distribution with effort distribution among the departments involved in the first-year curriculum for 1971–72. Comparisons are made of the various departments in terms of their percentage of total credit hours earned, percentage of total hours of direct contact with the students, percentage of faculty hours of contact with students as a percentage of total direct contact hours, and total department effort (direct contact with students plus preparation time) as a percentage of the total effort expended on the first-year curriculum.

There are some unusual variables reflected in these graphs. For example, Physiology-Pharmacology accounted for 25 percent of the total credit hours earned, 22 percent of the direct student contact, 14 percent of the faculty contact as a percentage of total contact, and 15 percent of the total de-

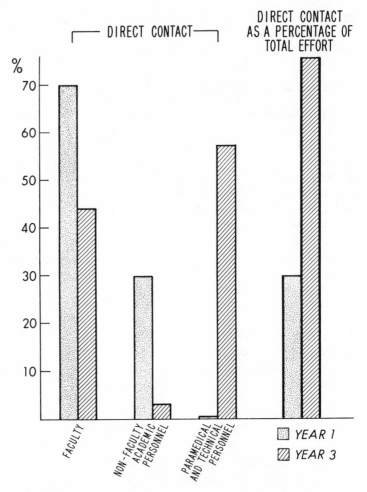

Figure XXVII–8. Comparison of total effort expended in the first and third curriculum years, 1971–72

partmental effort. The obvious disparity between credit-hour allocation and effort is even more clear in the case of Biochemistry where 19 percent of credit-hour allocation consumed only between 7 percent and 8 percent of direct contact, faculty contact, and total effort. Another pattern altogether is seen for Pathology, with 14 percent of credit hours earned, 26 percent of faculty contact, and 37 percent of total effort. Closer examination of these figures reveals that direct contact with students in Pathology is split almost evenly between faculty and residents or fellows. In Pathology, as well as Anatomy, the disparity between total departmental effort and credit-hour technical hours reported is necessary in preparation for the courses.

Although these graphs compare departmental expenditures of effort, an additional significant effort is made in the first years by the Central Teaching Facilities staff. No direct contact in a teaching mode is involved, but in terms of total effort this contribution constitutes 25.6 percent of all effort expended, mostly in support of courses in Biochemistry, Microbiology-Immunology, Physiology-Pharmacology, and Introduction to Clinical Diagnosis. This effort corresponds to the relatively higher number of hours in technical preparation which, because of the nature of intradepartmental programs, are required of the faculty in Anatomy and Pathology.

Figure XXVII–8 compared effort expended in the first and third years by three categories of personnel. The principal difference between these two years is in the percentage of direct contact with the student in terms of overall effort. In the first year, direct contact consumes 31 percent of the total departmental effort; in the third year it rises to 77 percent. However, in year one, 69 percent of this direct contact is by faculty, and 99 percent by a combination of faculty, house staff and graduate students. In the third year when the most effort is expended in direct contact with the student, only 44 percent of that contact is by faculty, with another 3 percent by non-faculty academic personnel. The remaining 53 percent of direct contact is by paramedical personnel, primarily advanced laboratory and medical technicians.

During 1971–72, the third-year credit-hour allocations were 47 percent to basic science department electives and 53 percent to nine special study programs. Analysis of the data on direct contact with the student and total hours of effort expended on third-year departmental electives and study programs showed that 61 percent of direct contact hours and 62 percent of the total hours of effort were expended by the basic science departments and that a significant proportion, 38 percent to 39 percent, of the total third-year effort was drawn from the clinical departments, most of it from the Department of Medicine. Only about half of this contribution was from faculty or other academic personnel, again confirming that a significant proportion of research preceptorship time is met by non-faculty personnel.

The second and fourth years, as noted above, are much more difficult to analyze. In both, it appears that contact with students consumes far more time than preparation for teaching. In the second year, this direct contact is split almost equally between faculty and non-faculty professionals (interns, residents, fellows). In the fourth year, the proportion of direct contact by faculty rises appreciably; where non-faculty professionals are utilized, they are usually senior residents or fellows.

Evaluation of Educational Programs

Every medical school that has experimented with curriculum revision has had difficulty in developing hard data regarding the effectiveness of the changes that were made. The faculty always starts to revise the curriculum with the expectation of improving the old system. Eventually the faculty must ask and answer these questions: "Does our curriculum adequately cover the material necessary for an understanding of the principles of modern medicine? Do the results of the new curriculum represent improvement over the old? Have we done a service or a disservice to our students?"

The answers to such questions are not easily come by. Superficially, it would appear that any school wishing to measure educational achievement could use an outside, well-established, presumably impartial review mechanism such as the National Board Examination. Closer consideration, however, reveals weaknesses in this approach. Curricula are tailored to the individual resources, students, faculty, traditions, aspirations, physical plant, and departmental strengths and weaknesses of a particular school, and presuppose time allocations to each discipline unique to that school. Finally, some schools use National Board scores in evaluating a student's fitness for promotion and graduation while other schools do not. For example, some schools "teach to the examination" while other schools, and Duke is included in this group, place no particular emphasis on doing well on these examinations. As a consequence, great care must be taken in comparing the scores of any one school's students with the national scores. This is particularly true when the changes in a particular curriculum are as extensive as those made at Duke. The National Board Examination, however, represents the best measuring mechanism available for what might be regarded as a national standard. Its tests are devised by panels of outstanding teachers and scientists in each of the basic and clinical disciplines; they are carefully constructed by experts in examining techniques.

Under the elective curriculum, our students were required to take Part I of the National Boards either in June or September following the freshman year. This arrangement was the one most favored by the students who felt they would be best prepared for the basic science examinations immediately following their classwork in these subjects. This procedure placed the Duke students at a minor disadvantage in terms of time allowed for assimilation of material, since the Boards presupposed two years of preparation rather than one.

Even with this handicap, the faculty believed it would be useful for our students to take Part I of the National Boards because the results might help gauge the effectiveness of the teaching of basic science at Duke against a national standard. A number of the responsible faculty felt that comparable performance on the tests would provide some assurance that we had identified the core areas of the basic sciences for teaching purposes.

Table XXVII−2 presents the average scores attained at Duke and nationally on Part I of the National Board Examination for five classes under the traditional curriculum and for the first five under the elective curriculum. During the first two years under the new curriculum, the average scores dropped 1.6 to 2.0 points, against both national averages and the records of students under the old curriculum. From 1972 through 1974, however, no significant differences appeared.

Table XXVII–2. National Board Examination, Part I: Average scores, Duke School of Medicine and national, 1962–67, 1969–74.

Exam year	M.D. year	Curriculum	Duke mean[a]	Nat. mean[b]
1962	1964	Traditional	79.3	80.3
1963	1965	,,	80.3	80.1
1964	1966	,,	81.3	80.6
1965	1967	,,	78.4	79.9
1966	1968	,,	82.3	80.9
1967	1969	,,	81.6	80.5
1969	1972	Elective	77.5	80.3
1970	1973	,,	78.3	80.3
1971	1974	,,	78.2	80.0
1972	1975	,,	80.0	80.1
1973	1976	,,	80.0	81.0
1974	1977	,,	82.0	81.0

a. Scores after one year of medical school.
b. Scores after two years of medical school.

The majority of Duke students take Part II of the National Boards at the end of their fourth year but they have the option of taking it any time after the second year. By the end of the fourth year the students have spent two years studying basic science and two years in clinical science. The actual time devoted to basic and clinical science is comparable to that spent under the old curriculum, but the material studied during these years is not comparable. Because early career decisions have influenced their choice of electives, almost every student has had curricular experience different from that of his classmates. Therefore, Duke students might seem to be at a disadvantage in national examinations devised to test students who have experienced more traditional curricula. When Part II test scores were analyzed, however, there was no significant difference between those of Duke students under the new curriculum and those under the traditional curriculum and both groups scored close to the national mean. Our students' experience with Part III of the National Board Examination was similar to that with Part II.

While our curriculum was undergoing revision, the National Board of Medical Examiners undertook to develop a series of examinations termed "Minitests" which were designed to evaluate the effect of curriculum change with respect to the pattern and extent of the student's learning. The Minitest

Table XXVII–3. Summary of Minitest scores, Medical School classes graduating 1969–75: basic science score clinical science score/total score

Year of graduation	Year test administered				
	Pre-Freshman	Freshman	Sophomore	Junior	Senior
1969 (Traditional Curriculum)	12.5 /3.8 /8.4.	33.3 /12.6 /24.1	46.8 /33.6 /40.9	43.28/40.30/41.98	42.42/42.96/42.76
1970 (Elective Curriculum)	18.0 /5.1 /12.3	43.3 /23.8 /34.5	37.23/37.20/37.20	41.32/36.42/39.34	40.95/41.64/41.31
1971 (Elective Curriculum)	16.7 /7.0 /12.3	38.72/24.42/32.17	38.80/36.30/37.93	43.31/41.60/42.63	45.00/46.68/45.64
1972 (E lective Curriculum)	15.18/9.78/12.73	40.45/19.20/30.91	41.26/39.23/40.40	41.51/38.44/40.01	40.70/46.72/43.52
1973 (Elective Curriculum)	15.05/4.37/10.25	39.53/23.69/32.27	43.22/39.38/41.33	42.66/45.14/43.87	43.68/42.32/42.90
1974 (Elective Curriculum)	13.58/8.53/11.31	40.32/24.15/32.72	40.40/41.98/41.15	42.36/39.86/41.08	42.10/45.33/43.60
1975 (Elective Curriculum)	15.16/7.03/11.30	40.09/28.07/34.59	41.50/39.83/40.63	41.86/43.39/42.64	Insufficient data

was made up of 360 pretested questions drawn from all twelve disciplines of Parts I and II of the regular National Board Examinations. The test was designed to be given in a single day. A new but equivalent form of the Minitest was created each year. All forms of the Minitest were matched in terms of medical content, based on category outlines as designated by the twelve basic and clinical science test committees of the National Board. Additional control was maintained by matching the various forms of the test in terms of difficulty (P value) and reliability. As designed, a single administration of the Minitest to all four classes in the spring, and then to the entering freshmen in the fall, would theoretically provide a cross-sectional view of five educational levels with respect to performance on the basic science sub-test. Further breakdown into first-year and second-year subjects and with respect to performance on the clinical science sub-tests also was possible. More important, from our point of view, was the opportunity provided by the tests to give information about patterns of learning in the old and new curricula.

The Minitest was administered to each entering class in the fall before the start of school and to the freshmen, sophomore, junior and senior classes, usually in the spring of the year. This meant that each class studied was given five Minitests. The test was given to the last class under the old curriculum (class of '69) and to the first five classes under the new curriculum. Every student was required to take an examination each year. The students were provided with information on the purpose and nature of these tests. They were not asked to make any special effort to prepare or review for the tests and they were assured that the tests would not be used in determining their class standing.

The mean scores are given in Table XXVII−3. The scores of "pre-freshmen" were essentially the same. In general, the results show no significant differences between the class under the traditional curriculum and the ones under the elective curriculum although there were a few variations in the time frame of the results which were undoubtedly related to the arrangement of the two curricula. The freshmen students who had completed one year of core basic science scores significantly higher in both basic and clinical science than the students who had spent one year in basic science under the traditional curriculum. This was attributed to the fact that the students had studied "core" material in all of the basic sciences under the elective curriculum and so had received a broader exposure than had students who had concentrated in anatomy, physiology and biochemistry under the pre-1966 curriculum. Then, too, the earlier group had not been exposed to microbiology, pharmacology, and pathology, subjects in which there is a fair degree of clinical correlation. On the other hand, when the sophomore basic science scores of the students who had had two years of basic science under the old curriculum were compared with the junior scores of the students after their elective year of basic science under the core curriculum, the scores showed no significant differences.

The most striking finding was that the average for both basic and clinical science for all years except the freshman and the mean score for both basic and clinical science for the senior classes were essentially the same.

On balance, the results from the National Board Examinations and the Minitests were comforting. Given the conditions described above, the faculty has generally been satisfied with these results, although higher scores would be welcome. At the very least, we have "done the patient no harm." The faculty apparently has succeeded in identifying a basic body of knowledge which enables our students to match the national average. More importantly, the scores demonstrate that the elective curriculum is broad enough to provide our graduates with a dependable body of medical knowledge which familiarizes them with the important phases of medicine essential to the understanding of disease processes in their patients and to discussion of their patients' problems with other physicians. At the same time, the flexibility of the elective curriculum frees the students from the shackles of a rigid schedule and permits them to make a stable, early career selection and to make use of a large and varied number of elective courses in preparation for it.

The attrition rate for students at Duke has traditionally been low. Great care always has been taken by the Admissions Committee to admit only students who were well qualified scholastically for the study of medicine. As a result, it is rare for a student to be asked to leave because of academic failure. The progress of each student is carefully monitored and when academic difficulties are encountered, various remedial steps are taken to help before the situation becomes too serious. Students who do fail courses are usually allowed to repeat or to do remedial work during the summer months if the Promotions Committee is convinced that the student truly desires to become a physician. Some students leave for personal reasons, usually because of a belated realization that they do not want to be physicians. Others transfer to other schools, either to follow a husband or wife or to be closer to parents. Still others transfer in order to work with a particular faculty member elsewhere.

For purposes of comparison, the attrition rates are given for the classes 1960–64 and 1970–74. Three students were dropped for academic difficulties during the years 1960–64 and only one during the years 1970–74. For the same periods, there were three transfers and nine withdrawals versus five transfers and eleven withdrawals. These differences are not significant (see Table XXVII–4).

Conclusion

Enrollment of students in a wide variety of basic science and clinical electives is an indication of student acceptance of the elective system and appreciation of its internal flexibility. It is rare for any two students in a given class to complete medical school with identical or even similar programs. The pressure exerted by the majority of students for direct clinical correla-

Table XXVII–4. Attrition among students in the Duke
University School of Medicine, 1960–65 and 1970–75

Entering class	Class size	Failure	Transfer	Withdrawals
1960–61	75	1	1	1
1961–62	76	0	0	2
1962–63	81	0	0	2
1963–64	82	2	2	3
1964–65	80	0	0	1
Total	394	3	3	9
1970–71	105	1	0	4
1971–72	105	0	2	1
1972–73	114	0	1	1
1973–74	114	0	2	3
1974–75	115	0	0	2
Total	553	1	5	11

tion of course content and the availability of alternative paths through the curriculum in preparation for a wide variety of medical careers provide the creative energy of the elective curriculum design.

The contributions of departments, individual faculty, and other health professionals to the total teaching effort are complex in their interrelationships and not readily measured by credit hours assigned for student performance. Similarly, the value of the elective curriculum is not easily measured by standardized tests, although test results do indicate no decrease in mastery of basic medical principles and information despite a radical decrease in required course hours. In the long run the capacity of this curriculum structure to generate physicians who can accommodate to future health system demands and technology and in so doing make significant contributions to meeting needs for medical care will determine the value assigned to the past decade of experience with the Duke curriculum.

XXVIII. Student Attitudes and Curriculum Change: A Longitudinal Study of Selected Variables

Jack J. Preiss, PH.D.

Robert A. Jackson, M.A.

Introduction

In 1961 the senior author of this chapter began a longitudinal study of Duke University medical students in order to examine the process of medical school training as it seemed to affect the developing self-image of the students. Beyond the substantive and technical aspects of training, the medical faculty were at that time interested in (1) the manner in which students made and altered career decisions, (2) student perceptions and evaluations of training, (3) the array of skills and abilities which students found important in training and early work; and (4) student attitudes toward the medical profession and patients. The chosen means for investigating these topics was a pretested questionnaire, covering a variety of attitudinal items, administered to each freshman class at entrance and again near the end of each academic year. This project began on the opening day of the 1961 fall term, and was intended to run for four years for each of three successive classes.

In 1963, two decisions were made which substantially altered the purpose and design of the study. First, the scope of the investigation was extended to include internship and residency years, since Duke students normally continue their formal training for several years beyond medical school. At the same time, the faculty entered into the planning of the elective curriculum, which is the subject of this book. Concurrently with the curriculum change, the faculty also agreed to a replication of the ongoing study with another set of three classes, trained under the new curriculum. This replication would permit some comparative analysis of the two curricula. In final form, then, the time format of the expanded design was as follows:

Table XXVIII–1. Chronological matrix of administration of questionnaires

	1961	'62	'63	'64	'65	'66	'67	'68	'69	'70	'71	'72	'73	'74	'75
Fixed Curriculum															
Class No. 1	Pre & 1st	2nd	3rd	4th	Int		Res								
Class No. 2		Pre & 1st	2nd	3rd	4th	Int		Res							
Class No. 3			Pre & 1st	2nd	3rd	4th	Int		Res						
Elective Curriculum															
Class No. 4							Pre & 1st	2nd	3rd	4th	Int		Res		
Class No. 5								Pre & 1st	2nd	3rd	4th	Int		Res	
Class No. 6									Pre & 1st	2nd	3rd	4th	Int		Res

Along with the potential for process analysis and the comparability of curricula provided by this format, some difficulties are also present. An obvious one is that since most Duke graduates take internships and residencies elsewhere, it is impossible to know how the non-Duke environments affect their attitudes during these years. In this regard, one simply records all the data without environmental differentiation.

A more technical issue concerns the statistical legitimacy of combining each set of three classes for a given year of training into a single unit in order to obtain a larger total number of cases (N) for analysis. To support this procedure, it was investigated and found that (1) admissions procedures were stable; (2) background characteristics, such as MCAT scores and socio-economic status, were similar; and (3) patterns of response on randomly selected questions were consistent. Under these circumstances, we felt that this combination of classes was legitimate.

Another typical problem with panel designs is loss of old respondents and additions of new ones from one time period to the next. In this study, losses were particularly noticeable in the advanced training years, primarily due to the necessity of mailing questionnaires. However, the rather impressive returns of between 60 and 70 percent for the mailed questionnaire, plus the random distribution of most intermittent losses (e.g., respondents failing to reply in one year, but doing so in subsequent years), convinced us that the panels were valid representatives of their curriculum groups.

Aside from these specific questions of structural design, the fifteen-year span of the study made it difficult to assess the impact of medical training of changes in American society during the 1960's. Many analysts have assumed or claimed that college students of this period were significantly more active and critical of American institutions than their predecessors of the 1950's. We are not able to measure the size of this difference, and it may, in retrospect, have been exaggerated by these analysts. Yet, we believe that major governmental innovations, such as Medicare, coupled with increasing public scrutiny of the medical profession in the mass media, have produced a heightened sensitivity to the larger society among medical students. Since we are not sure of the extent or effect of this changing climate on medical recruitment and training, we can only acknowledge its potential effect on student attitudes and encourage inquiry about it in future work.

We further recognize the possibility that the structure of the Duke program, and the findings to be presented concerning it, may not be representative of or applicable to other medical schools. Nevertheless, we feel that there are probably enough similarities among schools to make the experiences and analyses reported here at least partially relevant for a wide spectrum of schools at home and abroad.

Expression of medical career preferences

Since students anticipate their careers, and make decisions on the basis of their anticipations, even before entering medical school, this variable is

Table XXVIII-2. Medical career preference by training year

Training year	% general practice	% clinical speciali- zation	% academic medicine	% public health preventive medicine	% other	% undecided	% no answer	N
Fixed Curriculum								
Pretraining	11	46	10	—	—	32	—	235
First year	19	53	14	—	—	14	—	209
Second year	16	59	17	—	2	6	—	209
Third year	9	65	18	—	1	6	—	235
Fourth year	5	70	20	1	1	4	—	237
Internship	3	82	9	1	1	3	1	182
Residency	4	81	11	2	—	2	1	185
Elective Curriculum								
Pretraining	4	39	26	1	—	30	—	254
First year	6	40	28	2	—	24	—	252
Second year	7	55	25	2	1	10	—	244
Third year	4	64	22	2	—	5	3	243
Fourth year	6	68	21	1	1	1	1	208
Internship	7	71	14	2	2	4	—	136
Residency	6	71	18	1	2	1	—	150

*All of the tables in this chapter contain percentages rounded off to the nearest hundredth for ease of reading. This accounts for slight variations from 100% in the row totals. Such variations do not affect the validity of the analysis used in this discussion.

considered first. One of the stated goals of the new curriculum was to accelerate student expression of stable career preference choices so that students might elect advanced work, particularly in the third year, directly relevant to their ultimate professional goals. Clearly, given the pattern of rapid choice characteristic of students under the fixed curriculum (see Chapter I), the initial choice could not be accelerated very much.

As seen from Table XXVIII–2, the order and magnitude of career preference categories seems similar for both curricula. The dominant and central preference is "Clinical Specialization." Students entering since 1966 show a substantially greater initial interest in careers in academic medicine or research. Since increasing the Duke contribution to these career fields was another objective of the elective curriculum, these figures may indicate some success in attracting students in the desired categories. This interest wanes somewhat, however, to the point where, at the end of the fourth year, there appears little difference between the two groups. The interest among both groups also falls off sharply during internship, perhaps because of the dominant clinical orientation of the experience. However, recovery of the earlier academic orientation is stronger among elective curriculum students during their residencies. Also, since ten to twelve students in each class under the new curriculum entered combined M.D.–Ph.D. programs, thus slowing receipt of the questionnaires covering their internships and residencies, the final strength of the "Academic Medicine" category may be slightly greater than it appears here.

Some observers felt that an increase in public service and anti-specialization attitudes among college students in the 1960's would result in a substantial increase in the popularity of general practice and family medicine. The proportion of fixed curriculum students intending this career field at matriculation declined from the outset of their training, while under the elective curriculum a rather constant, low-level "General Practice" preference persists. Overall, while it may be too soon to gauge the full effect of the elective curriculum in changing the order of preference in careers, no alteration is yet visible. However, shifts may be underway which are more gradual and may emerge some years hence.

As expected, there is a steady and fairly rapid decline in indecision in both curricula. The greater delay in career choice during the first years of the elective curriculum may be attributable to the broader experience of students early in their training, which makes choice more difficult, or to the broader spectrum of career alternatives now available to graduate physicians, or to both. Table XXVIII–3 provides a picture of preference changes from year to year, both from one career preference to another and from decision to indecision.[1]

1. The data in this table were derived from a cross-tabulation of career preferences in pairs of consecutive years. Because the data are derived from paired responses, inclusion of cases is dependent upon availability of respondent questionnaires from both years of each consecutive pairing. Therefore, the reader will note that the N's of Table XXVIII–2 are discrepant with and

Table XXVIII–3. Components of career preference change by training stage and curriculum

Type of career preference change*	Training Stage					
	First year	Second year	Third year	Fourth year	Internship	Residency
Fixed curriculum						
Total N	206	177	191	221	172	150
Number and percentage of students indicating change	51(25)	41(23)	60(31)	50(23)	33(19)	20(13)
% Decided → undecided	29	12	18	10	12	10
% Clinical ↔ general practice	28	42	33	20	15	15
% Clinical ↔ academic medicine	37	34	38	54	58	16
% Other change	6	12	10	12	15	15
Elective curriculum						
Total N	251	235	219	188	114	99
Number and percentage of students indicating change	64(25)	60(26)	47(21)	23(12)	21(18)	18(18)
% Decided → undecided	44	13	11	9	19	6
%Clinical ↔ general practice	13	22	23	4	5	18
% Clinical ↔ academic medicine	33	52	60	74	67	56
% Other Change	11	13	6	13	10	22

*Single-headed arrows reflect one-way change: double-headed arrows indicate two-way change.

Three principal shift types account for more than 85 percent of career preference changes under either curriculum. Changes from a "Decided" to "Undecided" status[2] are most frequent in the first year, particularly of the elective curriculum, and decline in importance thereafter, as preconceptions are revised in light of actual training experiences. Such career preference change is again important in the third-year training period, when indecision

somewhat lower than those of other tables. This table presents (1) the principal components of career preference change, and (2) the proportion of students changing career preference during each training stage. Table XXVIII–3 portrays a complex phenomenon, the picture of which alters somewhat according to which factors of change are emphasized, so we caution the reader to keep in mind the possibility of alternative ways of summarizing the data.

2. The reader will note that this component describes only a one-way type of movement in contrast to the other components composed of two-way changes. The exclusion of those changing from "Undecided" to "Decided" omits students who, having indicated a career preference, are not expressing a real career preference change.

increases under the fixed curriculum, perhaps influenced by initial clinical experiences.

On a comparative basis, shifts between "General practice" and "Clinical specialization"[3] are more significant under the fixed curriculum, the larger percentage moving away from "General practice." Under the elective curriculum, where "General practice" is a more stable preference, the smaller flows of change approximately balance. In both curricula, shifts between "Academic medicine"[4] and "Clinical specialization" become increasingly important relative to other components. Under the fixed curriculum commitment to academic medicine increases from initially lower interest levels; the reverse is true under the elective curriculum. Other changes of career preference constitute a randomly distributed and small proportion of the total change occurring.

Under both curricula students tend to move either to "Clinical specialization" from "General practice" or "Academic medicine" or away from "Clinical specialization" toward one of the other two preferences. There is little movement between "General practice" and "Academic medicine," which are polar preferences. However, it is possible some such movement occurs involving an intermediate "Clinical specialization" preference through which movement between polar preferences is obscured. One difference to be noted is that "General practice" is a choice more widely considered under the fixed curriculum, whereas "Academic medicine" is, in the elective curriculum, much more involved in career choice deliberations. Another important difference is that, while approximately one student in four indicates change during the first two years of training under both curricula, the patterns diverge thereafter. During the third and fourth training years fixed curriculum respondents are more unresolved than their elective curriculum counterparts, suggesting that factors are operating under the elective curriculum which do promote career preference stability during the last half of undergraduate training.

Perceptions and evaluations of medical training

As in most professional training, medical education involves mastering a body of subject matter within a given setting—here the medical school and teaching hospital. This process is highly structured to facilitate learning and to monitor and react to performance. Intense relationships develop with faculty, patients and other students. All of this can be viewed as a total

---

3. The "Clinical Specialization" preference encompasses the entire range of specialty choice preference. Thus, in treating this as a unitary preference we are not looking at sub-levels of change in specialty choice (e.g., a change from surgery to pediatrics).

4. "Academic medicine" encompasses the alternatives of "Medical education," "Medical research," specialization within the academic setting, and various combinations thereof. For purposes of this discussion all of these preferences are treated as the single preference, "Academic medicine."

experience which students perceive and evaluate in different ways. The overall level of satisfaction with which students regard their training experiences is important both in itself, and as it bears on other aspects of the medical role, such as performance, career preference, and satisfaction with the decision to enter medicine. This section is limited to presentation and discussion of comparative curriculum findings concerning (1) student reactions to the training program as they judged it at the end of each training year and (2) the relationship of the "residency" judgment to satisfaction with the choice of a medical career.

The item from which training reactions are derived is elaborate and merits detailed discussion. The following question was asked at the end of each training year.[5]

> Select *two* of the following reactions which best characteristize your present *general* attitude toward *medical training*.
>
> | | | | |
> |---|---|---|---|
> | Boredom | Enthusiasm | Cynicism | Anger |
> | Uncertainty | Disillusionment | Dedication | Frustration |
> | Ambivalence | Disgust | Anxiety | Enjoyment |
>
> 1. Primary reaction _____
>   Chief reasons for selection:
> 2. Other important reaction _____
>   Chief reasons for selection:

Reduction of responses to manageable form first involves the preparation of summary tables for primary and secondary reactions separately. Both reactions are collapsed into three categories: positive, ambivalent and negative. "Uncertainty" and "Ambivalence" reactions comprise the ambivalent category. The other reactions, with the possible exception of "Boredom," are obviously positive or negative responses. "Boredom" verges on ambivalence but the connotation of weariness or tedium suggests passive dissatisfaction more than it does an equivocal attitude.[6]

The next step was to combine in reasonable fashion each respondent's primary and secondary reaction into an overall reaction toward training. To accomplish this, positive, ambivalent, and negative categories of the two reactions were paired in their nine possible combinations and arrayed on the scale shown below in Table XXVIII–4.[7]

5. In 1961 and 1962, the first two years of the study, the question was worded in slightly different fashion. The reactions "Anger" and "Frustration" were not included and respondents were not asked for a "primary" and "other" important reaction but instead for one or more reactions. Since most of these respondents gave only one reaction there are discrepancies in the N's of the first two pre-1966 curriculum training years in the tables to be presented.

6. The list of reactions is heavily weighted with negative adjectives (7 negative, 2 ambivalent, 3 positive) to which the reader might object. There is, however, a tendency to give positive responses to questions of this type. Inclusion of a disproportionate number of negative reactions is designed to overcome this response set and elicit more fully the degree of negativism actually experienced.

7. The particular scaling of combinations used here is achieved by double-weighting the primary response. By changing the weight of the primary with respect to the secondary response

Table XXVIII–4. Combination of primary and secondary reactions toward training categorization and index position of combined reactions*

Primary reaction	Categorization and index position of combined reactions*						
	Positive		Ambivalent			Negative	
	+3	+2	+1	0	−1	−2	−3
Positive	P/P	P/A	P/N				
Ambivalent			A/P	A/A	A/N		
Negative					N/P	N/A	N/N

*Combinations are notated with the primary reaction to the left of the slash and the secondary to the right.

Finally, the scale was partitioned into positive, ambivalent and negative categories. The two leftmost combinations were designated positive and the two rightmost negative, with the five intermediate combinations being ambivalent.

With the separate primary and secondary reactions an ambivalent response was the only way of expressing an equivocal attitude. In the combined reaction, however, a student is considered ambivalent (1) when his primary response is ambivalent or (2) when his separate responses are dissonant, that is, one negative and the other positive. The only difference between the primary and combined response distributions is that in the latter the ambivalent category expands at the expense of the positive and negative categories of the primary response distribution. The logic underlying this operational decision asserts that dissonance is actually another way of expressing ambivalence.

The partitioning tends to place most respondents into the ambivalent category. Only those clearly positive or negative in their combined reactions appear in the extreme categories.

This is the extent to which we transpose these data. No use is made in this presentation of the reasons respondents give for their reactions. These open-ended responses will become the subject of future analysis as satisfactory techniques are devised for cross-tabulation of them with the reaction categories.

Distributions of the primary, secondary and combined reactions toward medical training are sufficiently different in trend and apportionment to warrant separate presentation and discussion.

Table XXVIII–5 depicts the array of primary reactions for the entire training process.

---

the ordering of these combinations may be changed. It is left to the reader to decide whether we are introjecting the most defensible order on these data, keeping in mind that some type of weighting decision is necessary to derive a combined reaction.

Table XXVIII–5. Medical student distribution of primary reactions toward medical training by curriculum and training year

	Distribution by quality of primary reaction toward medical training				
Training year	% positive	% ambivalent	% negative	% other/no ans	N
Fixed curriculum					
First year	55	33	11	1	209
Second year	48	29	22	1	209
Third year	66	17	16	1	235
Fourth year	65	17	17	1	237
Internship	59	23	17	2	182
Residency	64	17	16	3	185
Elective curriculum					
First year	53	19	26	2	252
Second year	64	16	20	1	244
Third year	56	21	22	1	243
Fourth year	64	20	14	1	208
Internship	52	22	24	3	136
Residency	62	17	21	–	150

At the conclusion of all training years in both curricula the primary reaction is predominantly positive. The effect of time of introduction to clinical rotation is clearly evident. Negativism is greatest in the second year of the fixed curriculum with positive reactions rising to their peak in the third year. Contrastingly, clinical experience seems to improve satisfaction in the second year of the elective curriculum, an enthusiasm which dampens slightly the following year as students turn back to basic science material. In both curricula the level of satisfaction is relatively high in the fourth year, with a downward trend during the internship and a resurgence during the residency. The decline of enthusiasm during the new curriculum internship is steeper and recovery is less complete during the residency, with new curriculum residents ending up slightly less positive.

The perspective gleaned from Table XXVIII–5 changes in moving to consideration of findings for the secondary or "other important" responses. Negativism is a much larger component of secondary reaction in all stages of training. The responses of students under the fixed curriculum are marginally positive with a strong element of negativism most markedly expressed at the end of the second year of training. Secondary responses of students under the elective curriculum are marginally negative with a strong element of positive response.

There is more consistency in these responses from year to year than is apparent with the primary response. Among pre-1966 curriculum respondents the effect of clinical rotation in the third year is apparent, but not to the extent seen with the primary reaction. Interestingly, post-1966 curriculum respondents become less positive during the second year despite earlier introduction to clinical work. The pattern of "internship" responses in both

Table XXVIII-6. Medical student distribution of secondary reactions toward medical training by curriculum and training year

Training year	Distribution by quality of secondary reaction toward medical training				
	% positive	% ambivalent	% negative	% other/no ans	N
Fixed curriculum					
First year	47	13	33	7	76
Second year	44	7	44	5	133
Third year	45	20	34	2	235
Fourth year	47	16	34	3	237
Internship	44	11	39	7	182
Residency	48	13	31	9	185
Elective curriculum					
First year	44	10	41	5	252
Second year	38	18	41	4	244
Third year	40	13	40	8	243
Fourth year	38	15	44	4	208
Internship	36	12	46	7	136
Residency	41	10	43	6	150

curricula is not markedly different from the "fourth year" and "residency" responses, contrary to what is observed with primary reactions.

The unrelatedness of yearly trends in secondary reaction to clinical rotation and "internship" suggests these attitudes may reflect a set of concerns less tied to these experiences. The primary reaction appears sensitive to both the structure and process of medical training, while the secondary reaction seems less responsive to either of these aspects. One speculation holds that the student's secondary reaction is more often an evaluation of his performance in medical training and less an evaluation of the training itself; however, further investigation would be needed to bear this out. In short, it is rather unclear at this stage what secondary reactions mean (see Table XXVIII-6).

The results of the scaling and classification procedure previously described are reflected in the pattern of combined responses presented in Table XXVIII-7.[8] Ambivalence is the predominant element within the fixed curriculum with a strong secondary expression of satisfaction; in the elective curriculum ambivalence is more strongly expressed at the expense of satisfaction which, second year excepted, is well below that of the fixed curriculum. This stands in contrast to the patterns of primary response presented in Table XXVIII-5.

8. Since the primary and secondary reactions seem sensitive to different features of medical training experience, it might be suggested that combining the reactions is unwarranted. However, since Table XXVIII-7 is merely Table XXVIII-5 with students whose secondary reaction is polar to their primary reaction cast into the ambivalent category, the combined results bear examination because merging of the separate reactions is simple and because consideration of overall reaction to medical training is important.

Table XXVIII-7. Medical student distribution of combined primary and secondary reactions toward medical training by curriculum and training year

| Training year | Distribution by quality of combined reactions toward medical training | | | | |
	% positive	% ambivalent	%negative	% other/no ans	N
Fixed curriculum					
First year	37	50	8	5	95
Second year	26	60	10	4	154
Third year	45	43	10	3	235
Fourth year	42	45	9	4	237
Internship	31	52	9	7	182
Residency	41	41	10	9	185
Elective curriculum					
First year	27	57	10	6	252
Second year	34	53	9	4	244
Third year	29	52	11	8	243
Fourth year	33	55	8	5	208
Internship	23	55	15	7	136
Residency	35	47	12	6	150

The gap between the curricula on combined reactions stems from the differing extent to which dissonance is expressed. One of every four fixed curriculum students expresses it. Under the elective curriculum the ratio increases to one in three. By this measure, curriculum revisions may have lessened overall satisfaction with the program; certainly they do not appear to have produced appreciable or lasting improvement in it. However, caution must be exercised in interpreting these findings. The major portion of ambivalence expressed, especially under the elective curriculum, is of the dissonance variety. If we entertain the possibility that the positive aspect of this dissonance is primarily a response to the structure, demands, and quality of training and that the negative portion reflects a dissatisfaction with personal performance, then the apparent overall ambivalence would not be an indictment of the Duke curriculum as much as testimony to the inherent conflicts experienced by students engaged in a rigorous professional training process. Further investigation will hopefully clarify these matters.

One might expect students who are negative or ambivalent about their medical training to have serious reservations about having chosen a medical career. The findings presented in Table XXVIII-8 address this issue.

In this table the combined reactions of residents toward training are cross-tabulated against a judgment given by residents as to whether they would choose again to go through medical training knowing what they now know.[9] The results are enlightening. The principal finding, holding true for

9. In preparing Table XXVIII-8 several alternative ways of using training reactions were considered. Primary and secondary reactions were also tabulated against willingness to redo training; however, since the relationship was clearer and more consistent using the combined reaction, these other tables are not included.

Table XXVIII–8. Cross-tabulation of combined resident reactions toward medical training and willingness to redo training

Willingness to redo training	Combined resident reaction toward medical training				
	% positive	% ambivalent	% negative	% other/no ans	N
Fixed curriculum					
Yes	68	43	17	50	95
Probably, yes	26	45	50	50	71
Unsure	3	4	11	–	7
Probably, no	3	8	17	–	11
No	–	–	–	–	0
No Answer	–	–	6	–	1
N	76	75	18	16	185
Elective curriculum					
Yes	64	39	39	78	75
Probably, yes	31	51	39	22	61
Unsure	6	7	17	–	11
Probably, no	–	3	–	–	2
No	–	–	–	–	0
No Answer	–	–	6	–	1
N	52	71	18	9	150

both curricula, is that those expressing ambivalence or dissatisfaction toward training show little inclination to disavow their earlier choice of medicine as an occupation. No student indicates with certainty he would not choose medicine again. A small percentage under the fixed curriculum and a negligible number under the elective curriculum indicate they probably would not choose medicine again. The "Unsure" category is small in both curricula. The certain and uncertain "Yes" groups make up the overwhelming majority of students. To the extent a relationship exists between training reaction and appropriateness of occupational choice it is found in the narrow range of affirmativeness in that those ambivalent or negative toward training are more likely to indicate, "Probably, yes."

Since most students would probably choose medicine again regardless of their reactions toward training, the meaning of attitudes toward training is further obscured. If one views medical training as a difficult and prolonged initiation process, then presumably the more suffering and effort required of the student the more meaningful the goal of achieving full professional status becomes. This sort of cognitive dissonance explanation would account for the fact that under the elective curriculum less favorable attitudes toward training seem to result in even greater attachment to the medical profession choice. In this view, reactions to training are largely a form of ventilation engaged in by medical students under great pressure.

A complementary and more deterministic view might be to suggest that an entrapment process is occurring. Achieving the M.D. degree is a cherished

Table XXVIII–9. Percentage of students viewing selected skills and competencies as important in getting the most out of training experiences

	Technical		Informational		Behavioral			
	1	2	3	4	5	6	7	
Training year	Manual dexterity	Memorization ability	Natural science knowledge	Social science knowledge	Getting along with other students or colleagues	Making up your mind about study emphasis	Ability to participate in research	N
Fixed curriculum								
Pretraining	69	95	83	23	89	93	44	235
First year	26	96	85	35	80	93	18	209
Second year	40	98	67	23	71	88	11	209
Third year	49	88	68	21	77	90	19	235
Fourth year	58	87	63	27	71	90	17	237
Internship	75	55	63	36	84	71	8	182
Residency	57	57	60	41	79	83	28	185
Elective curriculum								
Pretraining	55	91	78	28	88	93	38	254
First year	29	94	84	16	77	87	10	252
Second year	61	79	65	25	83	90	10	244
Third year	23	59	72	21	70	93	51	243
Fourth year	46	65	65	30	72	92	20	208
Internship	77	47	57	40	73	62	2	135
Residency	62	58	61	52	89	88	13	150

Type of skill or competence

goal for those allowed to undertake the journey. No other profession offers better guarantees of financial security and esteem. In order to achieve this goal, however, unremitting personal sacrifice is required of the M.D. candidate. A commitment is developed toward a high-status occupation which, if reneged upon, leads to no alternatives of equal status. Even if the student finds medical training abhorrent and the prospect of practice unappealing, it is difficult to acknowledge misdirection in one's life work. To seriously admit other more compelling career interests would be to become a less estimable person in the eyes of many.

Skills, abilities and techniques

Medical education is, in one important sense, a process of developing a number of skills and competencies which directly affect the acquisition and implementation of medical knowledge. A variety of techniques and formats are utilized in both academic and practical courses. This study attempted to chart the ebb and flow of these patterns throughout the training program. Each year the students were asked to rate the importance of a fixed number of skills and competencies. By using a stable group of factors covering a diversity of types it was possible to see shifts of emphasis in how students evaluated their learning experiences, and how they perceived some of the capabilities they were trying to acquire.

Table XXVIII–9 shows the relatively high level of importance attached to the entire range of factors by the pretraining students. This is true in a rather consistent pattern of emphasis in both curricula, and may be explained as a typical expression of both anxiety and uncertainty of students embarking on a rigorous professional program. During the training year the technical skills, manual dexterity and memorization ability are felt to be of less importance by undergraduates under the elective curriculum, but reacquire comparable levels of importance during the internship and residency years, when a majority of respondents are no longer at Duke. Natural science knowledge is very highly valued under both curricula, while the importance of social science knowledge increases more rapidly in the graduate training years among students who studied under the elective curriculum. Since the rate of increase in importance of this type of information is most dramatic after Duke students have dispersed to other institutions, one might hypothesize that the value attached to this item is more a part of the current "atmosphere" within the profession than the product of purposive educational procedures in one medical school. This, of course, is a speculative judgment requiring further investigation.

Items five and six show the least variability over time, and are obviously seen by the students in both curricula as the most important items among all of those presented, exceeding both technical and informational factors by a rather impressive margin. This may suggest that the *way* one works is seen as generally a more important category in the training process than one's innate talents or intellectual resources. Again, curriculum changes have not appeared to affect the relative importance of these types, a finding consistent with the non-curricular nature of the behavioral factors.

Since one objective of the elective curriculum is to prepare students more adequately for careers in medical research, it is significant that students trained under the elective curriculum generally do not regard the ability to participate in research as being of major importance. There is strong student response in the third year of the elective curriculum, when research is most highly emphasized, but this stimulus apparently is short-lived. Cross-tabulations of career preference and the ability to participate in research (not presented in this article) reveal that in any given year of either curriculum the clinical specialist was just as likely to find this item important as was the student choosing academic medicine as a career preference. This suggests that the item is sensitive to the specific demands of the training situation rather than to strongly or weakly developed research orientations among the majority of students. As medical graduates disperse into internships and residencies there is little indication that they are moving into situations where research ability again is emphasized. The implication would seem that promoting research orientations among medical students in part depends upon consistent opportunities and encouragement to participate in research. These are perhaps not being made widely available to students beyond the undergraduate years.

Finally, students were asked throughout their training to assess their relative effectiveness in patient care. Table XXVIII–10 presents the results. The most notable feature is their uniformity, showing perhaps the least variation of any variable in the study. Despite numerous changes by individuals rating themselves from year to year, the net change from pretraining to residency was negligible. Since about 50 percent of the responses in any given year fall into the equality-of-skills category and about 25 percent into each of the polar preferences, students may be reflecting a bias toward the central category because of the connotation it implies of the well-rounded physician.

Methods of training

Closely related to skills, abilities and techniques, are the methods employed to teach them. The predominantly "straight" academic years (first and second in the fixed curriculum; first and third in the elective curriculum) followed typical classroom laboratory teaching patterns. More variety was found in the clinical rotations and the advanced years. Since students usually felt most significant medical training was concentrated in clinical settings, it seemed logical to examine the learning patterns used in those settings. There were four principal methods—rounds, conferences, seminars and independent reading. Each is examined with respect to student evaluation of its effectiveness, as expressed in open-ended responses concerning the method.

Table XXVIII–10. Student self-evaluations of patient care skills

Training year	% physical diagnosis and treatment	% equal skill in both areas	% interpersonal aspects of patient care	% no answer	N
Fixed curriculum					
Pretraining	31	45	23	1	235
First year	25	52	23	—	209
Second year	27	53	19	2	209
Third year	28	48	24	—	235
Fourth year	23	54	22	1	237
Internship	27	53	18	2	182
Residency	28	46	23	3	185
Elective curriculum					
Pretraining	30	47	22	1	254
First year	23	54	23	1	252
Second year	24	45	31	1	244
Third year	22	49	27	2	243
Fourth year	18	54	28	1	207
Internship	23	55	21	1	136
Residency	28	47	23	2	150

Table XXVIII–11. Evaluation of rounds

	% clear positive	% moderate or qualified positive	% clear negative	% not evaluated or other	N
Fixed curriculum					
Third year*	37	48	2	13	235
Fourth year	31	63	4	2	237
Internship	30	41	13	16	182
Residency	24	29	11	36	185
Elective curriculum					
Second year*	21	62	12	5	244
Fourth year	31	33	13	23	208
Internship	15	46	15	24	136
Residency	15	31	13	41	150

*These two years are experience equivalents, since the initial clinical year was shifted to the second year in the elective curriculum.

Rounds are probably the most distinctive and glamorized of medical teaching devices. They are inclined to receive a qualified positive response from many students, and in several of the years a considerable number make no evaluative comments. In the qualified responses, the major variable is the rounding staff person, in that students judge some to be markedly inferior to others. Undergraduate students responded to rounds more positively under the fixed curriculum than did those under the elective (see Table XXVIII–11).

Table XXVIII–12. Evaluation of conferences

	% clear positive	% mixed	% clear negative	% not evaluated or other	N
Fixed curriculum					
Third year	11	54	5	30	235
Fourth year	19	67	8	6	236
Internship	24	41	16	19	182
Residency	30	32	10	28	185
Elective curriculum					
Second year	26	48	13	13	244
Fourth year	30	34	7	29	208
Internship	19	42	14	25	136
Residency	31	35	11	23	150

Conferences usually take the form of patient presentations, live and with other visual aids, in a large room with substantial numbers of students present. Student involvement is more as observer than participant, though participation increases in the advanced years. Table XXVIII–12 shows a consistently higher positive than negative evaluation in both curricula, with the internal patterns of each rather similar. In some years, the "mixed" category equals the combined total of the positive and negative types. It is difficult to discern any definitive trends in these distributions, and it seems safe to say only that conferences are usually judged to be an acceptable format for training, with only minor differences between curricula.

Compared with "Rounds," under the curricula in the two undergraduate clinical years the positive view of conferences is noticeably stronger in the elective curriculum. After the majority of students move elsewhere for advanced training, the profiles of the two curriculum groups become much alike.

Table XXVIII–13. Evaluation of seminars

	% clear positive	% mixed	% infrequent use	% clear negative	%not evaluated or other	N
Fixed curriculum						
Third year	11	12	23	8	46	235
Fourth year	9	11	48	13	19	237
Internship	4	8	49	12	27	182
Residency	22	8	22	11	37	185
Elective curriculum						
Second year	26	27	20	11	16	244
Fourth year	23	13	16	8	40	208
Internship	4	8	36	10	42	136
Residency	15	22	15	12	35	150

The data in Table XXVIII – 13 indicate that seminars are considerably less used than other methods. Often, fewer than one half the students have any evaluation of this method, and negative views sometimes are more prominent. No linear trends emerge in chronological terms. The same pattern can be seen as was observed regarding "Conferences." The clinical years indicate more positive acceptance of seminars in the elective curriculum, but the curriculum group differences disappear in the advanced training years, after most of the students have left Duke for other schools and hospitals.

Table XXVIII–14. Evaluation of independent reading

	% clear positive	% qualified positive	% lack of time	% clear negative	% not evaluated or other	N
Fixed curriculum						
Third year	30	18	31	0	31	235
Fourth year	46	19	20	2	13	237
Internship	28	6	41	2	21	182
Residency	47	10	19	1	23	185
Elective curriculum						
Second year	35	12	41	2	11	244
Fourth year	51	6	11	2	30	208
Internship	15	4	49	3	29	136
Residency	46	6	27	1	19	150

While it may come as no surprise to those who have been continually engaged in medical education, it is quite clear from Table XXVIII – 14 that independent reading is the primary positive method of medical education in the eyes of medical students in both curricula, and in almost exactly the same magnitude. The "Intern" distributions are interesting because they suggest that this year is characterized by considerable frustration at not being able to read as much as is desired. Thus, the low level of "Clear Positive" for this year should not be interpreted as a decline in the value of reading in one's own, but only the lack of time to do it. The "Residency" indicates a return to the relative distributions of the clinical years.

Approval for independent reading is much greater than for other methods, although its use is sometimes limited by other demands on time and energy. This finding suggests that perhaps the most effective thing a curriculum change can provide is simply more free time for students to work on their own. This does not mean total lack of direction or accountability. But it does suggest that students regard their own learning to be enhanced more by this method than any other. If such is actually true, medical schools might well consider not only the improved learning possible for students with more recognition (and time made available) for this method, but the concomitant savings to be gained in staff time, facilities, and similar resources.

Differences in expectations

In any education program, there are individual experiences and reactions which are unanticipated by the students. Such experiences and reactions are best gathered by giving students the opportunity to identify them in an open-minded manner. This precludes any control of responses by forced choice or selected topics. The price the investigator pays for allowing this free choice by respondents is a diversity of answers in which it is often difficult to achieve a manageable number of foci for analysis. The complexity of the data was compounded by the fact that respondents were not limited in this survey as to the number of factors or experiences they could specify. This sometimes resulted in a situation in which number of mentions differed widely from the number of respondents. For example, if one respondent mentioned five factors and four mentioned none, simple addition would give five mentions and five people without any inkling of how the five mentions actually were distributed. Although the "No Answer" rate was well under 10 percent throughout the fixed curriculum, it reached almost 18 percent in the third year of the elective curriculum.

It was decided to limit the tabulated factors to a maximum of three. The reasons were (1) the data presentation became unwieldy for larger numbers and (2) less than one-half the respondents gave more than two factors. The major precaution against response bias in this section of the survey was to assure the student (as part of the question) that positive as well as negative material was sought. A summary of these responses is displayed in Table XXVIII–15.

Table XXVIII–15. Aspects of medicine and medical training different from expectations

Training year	% nothing different	% positive	% negative	ambiguous	% no answer or no other mentions	N
Fixed curriculum						
First year						
1st mention	7	39	39	13	2	209
2nd mention	7	26	33	5	29	209
3rd mention	7	14	15	4	60	209
Second year						
1st mention	10	19	58	11	3	209
2nd mention	10	19	25	10	36	209
3rd mention	10	9	11	3	68	209
Third year						
1st mention	14	24	45	14	3	235
2nd mention	14	16	30	6	34	235
3rd mention	14	8	15	3	60	235

Fourth year						
1st mention	12	21	40	19	8	237
2nd mention	12	16	25	11	36	237
3rd mention	12	8	10	7	64	237
Internship						
1st mention	16	9	48	20	8	182
2nd mention	16	7	30	10	37	182
3rd mention	16	4	13	6	62	182
Residency						
1st mention	14	13	44	30	9	185
2nd mention	14	15	24	16	31	185
3rd mention	14	3	10	9	64	185
Elective curriculum						
First year						
1st mention	9	22	40	24	5	252
2nd mention	9	20	30	17	24	252
3rd mention	9	14	21	6	50	252
Second year						
1st mention	9	21	39	26	5	244
2nd mention	9	22	23	21	24	244
3rd mention	9	11	13	9	57	244
Third year						
1st mention	11	23	34	15	18	243
2nd mention	11	16	21	8	44	243
3rd mention	11	5	10	3	71	243
Fourth year						
1st mention	12	25	31	20	12	208
2nd mention	12	13	22	6	47	208
3rd mention	12	5	11	2	69	208
Internship						
1st mention	7	17	54	10	13	136
2nd mention	7	10	43	8	32	136
3rd mention	7	6	19	4	64	136
Residency						
1st mention	7	17	47	19	9	150
2nd mention	7	12	31	17	33	150
3rd mention	7	7	11	5	70	150

Few students had no unexpected experiences. Unexpected experiences usually were valued negatively. Students under the fixed curriculum were more critical of the undergraduate training period than students under the elective curriculum. However, they were less critical of the advanced training period when many were at institutions other than Duke. Students trained under the elective curriculum were markedly more negative toward unexpected experiences in the internship and residency periods than when they were in medical school at Duke. What is being reflected in the category of

"Negative Surprise" indicated by these figures is not clear, although the category was present for most students under both curricula.

The kind of surprise most frequently cited included responses to one or more aspects of the training process. Table XXVIII – 16 indicates that students under the fixed curriculum more frequently experienced negative surprise during the training process than students following the elective pattern. The markedly higher ratio of negative to positive responses in the advanced training years also is noteworthy.

Table XXVIII–16. Differences from expectations related to the training process: frequency and quality of mentions by curriculum and training year

Training year	Frequency and quality of mentions				
	No. positive	No. negative	No. ambiguous	No. mentions*	Total N †
Fixed curriculum					
First year	75	94	29	198	209
Second year	33	100	22	155	209
Third year	55	117	28	200	235
Fourth year	40	74	30	144	237
Internship	7	49	11	67	182
Residency	9	24	9	42	185
Elective curriculum					
First year	42	97	54	193	252
Second year	49	63	49	161	244
Third year	50	52	31	133	243
Fourth year	39	45	21	105	208
Internship	11	37	5	53	136
Residency	8	27	11	46	150

*Represents the total number of 1st, 2nd and 3rd mentions in any given year.
†Represents the number of respondents from which the mentions were obtained.

The relationships of students to senior staff vary considerably from year to year, ranging from formal contact in academic settings to sporadic or intensely personal contact in clinical situations. The experiences of the two curricular groups in terms of this variable were strikingly similar. If the curricular shift did produce notable changes in the training program, this was not reflected in the quantity or quality of unexpected experiences with faculty as reported by the students (see Table XXVIII – 17).

Experiences different from expectations with respect to the medical profession generally and medical careers in general were only infrequently reported during the first three training years by students under the fixed curriculum. Thereafter, however, they were mentioned often. Mentions by students under the elective curriculum are more evenly distributed across the training period; however, mentions are proportionately more frequent during graduate training. As with the two substantive variables just dis-

Table XXVIII–17. Differences from expectations of relations with the senior staff or faculty: frequency and quality of mentions by curriculum and training year

Training year	Frequency and quality of mentions				
	No. positive	No. negative	No. ambiguous	No. mentions*	Total N †
Fixed curriculum					
First year	32	30	1	63	209
Second year	23	34	8	65	209
Third year	17	38	2	57	235
Fourth year	15	41	6	62	237
Internship	2	20	4	26	182
Residency	1	11	2	13	185
Elective curriculum					
First year	35	37	13	85	252
Second year	26	43	12	81	244
Third year	15	33	5	53	243
Fourth year	11	24	4	39	208
Internship	6	21	0	27	136
Residency	2	30	5	37	150

*Represents the total number of 1st, 2nd and 3rd mentions in any given year.
†Represents the number of respondents from which the mentions were obtained.

Table XXVIII–18. Differences from expectations related to the medical profession and a medical career: frequency and quality of mentions by curriculum and training year

Training year	Frequency and quality of mentions				
	No. positive	No. negative	No. ambiguous	No. mentions*	Total N †
Fixed curriculum					
First year	2	0	1	3	209
Second year	2	3	4	9	209
Third year	8	7	7	22	235
Fourth year	8	15	21	44	237
Internship	9	46	30	85	182
Residency	23	53	31	107	185
Elective curriculum					
First year	5	6	12	23	252
Second year	8	22	17	47	244
Third year	5	16	8	29	243
Fourth year	6	16	11	33	208
Internship	5	27	8	40	136
Residency	12	20	7	39	150

Represents the total number of 1st, 2nd and 3rd mentions in any given year.
†Represents the number of respondents from which the mentions were obtained.

cussed above, the reactions of students were dominantly negative toward unexpected experience (see Table XXVIII – 18).

In summary, investigation of student attitudes toward unexpected experiences reveals surprisingly uniform response patterns, whether toward single substantive variables or between curricula. Although most students had training experiences which differed from their expectations and which they valued negatively, apparently these were not severe or frequent enough to divert them to other careers. In short, they coped. The persistence of these unexpected experiences suggests that changes in the formal curriculum have little effect on those aspects of training to which such experiences are related.

Attitudes of Graduate Physicians Toward Training, the Profession, and Patients

By the time students completed the fourth year of training they had accumulated sufficient experience with medicine to formulate attitudes concerning the major areas of concern: training, patients, and the medical profession itself. Accordingly, a set of statements designed to tap attitudes in these three areas was attached to the last three questionnaires administered to each student. Available time and space precluded asking a large number of questions pertinent to each area; the analysis which follows is based upon responses to the three questions in each area which proved to be most definitive as attitude indicators. The students used a Likert-type scale of response, with two levels of agreement and two of disagreement from which to choose.

Simple tests reveal no statistically significant differences between the two curriculum groups. Indeed, since these questions were asked primarily of students in the internship and residency years, the responses are much more closely related to the original project purpose—that is, to measuring the relationship of training to student self-image—than to any comparison of curricula. They are offered, however, because they may illuminate implications of the data presented earlier.

Figure XXVIII – 1 indicates that student attitudes toward training, marginally more positive at the end of the fourth year of training under the elective curriculum, are marginally more negative after the internship and residency years. All of the means are grouped near the mid-point of the negative-positive scale. Reponses are scaled from strongly negative (SN) through moderately negative (MN) and moderately positive (MP), to strongly positive (SP).

Student attitudes toward patients similarly center at the midpoint of the attitude scale. Students under the elective curriculum have marginally more positive attitudes toward patients in each of the three years (see Figure XXVIII – 2).

Neither does curriculum change appear to have affected appreciably the attitude of students toward the medical profession. But, more important than

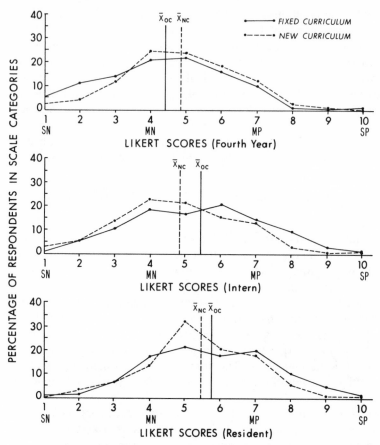

Figure XXVIII–1. Distribution of fourth year, intern, and resident responses on Likert training items by curriculum

a curricular comparison, students frequently are negative toward the profession generally. The tendency is somewhat more pronounced among the elective curriculum group and, for that group, becomes particularly apparent during the intern year (see Figure XXVIII–3). This finding adds weight to the conclusion that elective curriculum students are more critical of the profession than they are of the individual facets of training or the training process overall. This may reflect the increasing restiveness of Americans over the issue of the availability of quality health care and perhaps accounts, in part, for the dissonance mentioned above in connection with responses to training.

Review of these three attitude-areas as a group reveals a general similarity of student attitude-patterns under the two curricula, with little change during the advanced years of training and a marginally negative attitude-set toward the profession of medicine in its broadest context. These findings do not

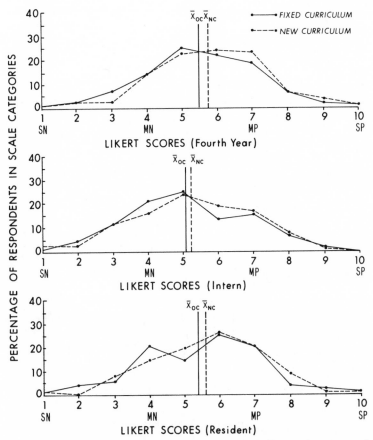

Figure XXVIII–2. Distribution of fourth year, intern, and resident responses on Likert patient items by curriculum

mean that medical students are dissatisfied with their chosen careers or that they perform poorly in them; indeed, a certain amount of dissatisfaction is probably healthy during the training period because it opens the way for constructive change. Nevertheless, the findings might mean that changes in the undergraduate curriculum do not, of themselves, sustain positive attitudes among medical students toward training and practice. If such attitudes are desired, it is clearly necessary now to investigate further the interface between undergraduate and graduate medical education. We must also carefully scrutinize several areas outside the formal medical education framework. Included among these are the process by which students are recruited, the current organizational flux within the medical profession, and the political and legislative processes which increasingly have affected medical practice in recent years.

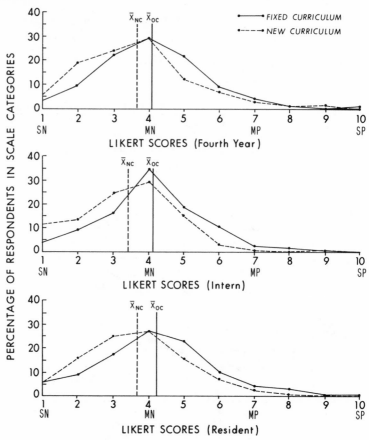

Figure XXVIII–3. Distribution of fourth year, intern, and resident responses on Likert profession items by curriculum

XXIX. The Graduates

William D. Bradford, M.D.

Charles B. Johnson, ED.D.

Thomas D. Kinney, M.D.

Introduction

In this chapter we compare the five medical school classes that graduated in the years 1960–64 with the five classes graduating in the years 1970–74. The classes from 1965 through 1969 are not included because this was the transition period from the traditional four-year curriculum to the elective curriculum. The classes of 1960–64 and 1970–74 are compared with regard to number, sex, race, geographic origin by region and state, rank order success in the National Intern and Resident Matching Program, internships by medical center and specialty, and number entering primary care. In addition, a summary of our experience with curriculum acceleration and with the early internship program is presented. This information will become more precise and useful when in later years we look at the 1970–74 graduates in terms of residency training, practice specialty and geographic location.

Number and origins of graduates

The total number of students graduating in the years 1970–74 exceeded by forty the number who graduated in 1960–64 due to growth in class size during the late 1960's, but this does not take into account the fact that in 1972 the number of admissions was increased to 114. The average class size of the 1960 period was 79 members; that of the 1970 period 87. Females comprised only 2 percent of the classes during 1960–64 but comprised 10 percent of each class during 1970–74. The average size of the classes graduating in 1978 and 1979 will be approximately 114, and approximately 27 percent will be women (see Table XXIX–1).

When the graduates are considered in relation to their geographic origin as listed at time of admission, several differences are evident between the 1960 and 1970 groups. These differences no doubt reflect changes in the selection process. In the 1960–64 groups, 266 students (66.5 percent) came from the South Atlantic states, 64 (16 percent) from the Middle Atlantic, and 30 (9.5 percent) from the South Central. Only 6 or (1.5 percent) claimed New

Table XXIX–1. Number of graduates by sex and race

Graduates	1960	1961	1962	1963	1964	Total	1970	1971	1972	1973	1974	Total
Male	74	79	78	78	84	393	61	70	86	85	91	394
Female	2	2	1	1	1	7	9	10	12	5	10	45
Total	76	81	79	79	85	400	70	80	98	91	101	440
Caucasian	75	81	77	78	85	396	70	79	97	87	95	428
Black								1		3	6	10
Oriental				1		1			1	1		2
Spanish SN	1		2			3						
Total	76	81	79	79	85	400	70	80	98	91	101	440

England as their permanent residence. The graduating students of the 1970–74 period were more evenly distributed with 203 (46 percent) from the South Atlantic states, 102 (23 percent) from the Mid-Atlantic, and 30 (9 percent) from the South Central. More students also were selected from the Middle Atlantic, New England, North Central and Pacific regions in the 1970's (see Table XXIX–2).

When representation from individual states is considered, North Carolina clearly has more representatives in both study groups than any other state. However, during the period 1970–74, the number of graduates from North

Table XXIX–2. The number of graduates by geographic area

Geographic area	Total 1960–64	%	Total 1970–74	%
South Atlantic	266	66.50	203	46.14
Middle Atlantic	64	16.00	102	23.18
South Central	30	7.50	39	8.86
North Central	18	4.50	38	8.63
New England	6	1.50	29	6.59
Pacific	7	1.75	14	3.18
Mountain	5	1.25	11	2.50
Foreign	4	1.00	4	0.91
Total	400	100	440	100

Table XXIX–3. Graduates by state of residence on admission

1960–64			1970–74		
State	Number	% Total	State	Number	% Total
North Carolina	130	32.50	North Carolina	78	17.72
Florida	40	10.00	New York	50	11.36
New York	30	7.50	Virginia	32	7.27
Virginia	27	6.75	Florida	25	5.68
South Carolina	25	6.25	New Jersey	29	6.59
New Jersey	23	5.75	Pennsylvania	23	5.22
Georgia	18	4.50	Maryland	23	5.22
West Virginia	15	3.75	Tennessee	18	4.09
Pennsylvania	11	2.75	Georgia	17	3.86
Other U.S.	77	19.25	Connecticut	14	3.18
Foreign	4	1.00	South Carolina	14	3.18
Total	400	100	Ohio	13	2.95
			Massachusetts	12	2.72
			California	12	2.72
			West Virginia	10	2.27
			Other U.S.	66	15.00
			Foreign	4	0.91
			Total	440	100

Table XXIX–4. The graduates and the National Intern Matching Plan

Class of	1960–64						1970–74					
	1960	1961	1962	1963	1964	Total	1970	1971	1972	1973	1974	Total
Total graduates	76	81	79	79	85	400	70	80	98	91	101	440
No. participants NIMP	57	64	65	67	71	324	64	59	67	65	65	320
% participants	75	79	82	85	84	81	92	74	68	72	64	73
No. non-participants	19	17	14	12	14	76	6	21	31	26	36	120
% non-participants	25	21	18	15	16	19	8	26	32	28	36	27

Matching by rank order

Rank order	1960	1961	1962	1963	1964	Total	%	1970	1971	1972	1973	1974	Total	%
1	39	53	46	40	50	228	70	36	33	42	32	35	178	56
2	6	6	6	11	11	40	12	14	11	12	7	13	57	18
3	5	2	6	4	5	22	7	3	6	6	4	4	23	7
4	2	1	2	4	4	13	4	5	3	2	3	6	19	6
5	2	1	0	6	1	10	3	1	3	1	6	2	13	4
6	1	1	0	1	0	3	1	0	1	1	2	3	7	2
7	2	0	0	0	0	2	0.6	1	0	0	0	0	1	0.3
8	0	0	0	0	0	0	0	4	2	3	0	1	10	3
Unmatched participants	0	1	5	1	0	7	2	4	2	3	8	1	18	6

Carolina decreased while the number of graduates from other states, especially New York, increased. This increase is a temporary one, for the number of North Carolina students has increased markedly since 1969, when the state instituted a scholarship plan to support North Carolina residents in private medical schools. Table XXIX–3 describes this experience.

The graduates and the matching plan

Eighty-nine percent of the Duke graduates participating in the National Intern and Resident Matching Program from 1960–65 matched with one of their first three choices. Seven students were not matched initially during these years. It should be noted that failure to match is not necessarily a reflection of the individual student's record and potential. Often unmatched students obtain stronger positions than matched students by being on the "open market" after the matching process. The data from the classes of 1970–75 show that 81 percent of this group matched with one of their first three choices. Eighteen students (6 percent of the entire group) were intially unmatched.

Seventy percent of the 1960's group matched with their first choice, while 56 percent of the 1970's group did so. The 26 percent decrease in successful matching with first choice could be explained in part by the fact that more of our students are seeking postgraduate training in nationally prominent and competitive programs (Table XXIX–4). Another possible reason for the decrease is that 27 percent of the 1970's study group were *non*-participants in the NIMP because they graduated early and entered postgraduate programs of their own choosing. This is an important trend to follow. As more medical schools evolve flexible curricula and more students move at their chosen pace, an increasing number of graduates will finish at various times during the year. It is quite likely that in the future it will be necessary for postgraduate programs to recognize this increasing variability in the dates of graduation.

"Early Graduation"—the effects of acceleration

Duke traditionally has made it possible for its students to complete the required four academic years in less calendar time. Since the late 1960's, over 50 percent of each medical school class has completed requirements for the M.D. degree prior to the traditional spring commencement.

Seventy students (67 percent) of the class of 1975 accelerated their completion of the requirements for the M.D. degree. Of these early graduates, twenty-seven (39 percent) did not enter, or withdrew from the National Intern Matching Program prior to the matching process. Of these twenty-seven, fourteen interned at Duke, three in the U.S. Military services, two at Cornell, and one each at Yale, The University of Washington, Vanderbilt,

Johns Hopkins, and North Carolina. Clearly these early graduates from the class of 1975 were able to negotiate strong postgraduate training slots without the aid of the matching plan (see Table XXIX–5).

Table XXIX–5. Acceleration in the curriculum: Duke Medical School graduates, 1970–75

	1970	1971	1972	1973	1974	1975
Total number of graduates	70	80	98	91	101	104
Early graduates	27	39	53	48	62	70
Percent of class as early graduates	38	48	54	53	61	67

The early internship program

Some students have chosen to establish a more direct continuity between medical school and postgraduate training by merging the fourth year of medical school and the traditional internship. Beginning in 1971, this opportunity was offered to students with outstanding academic records. These students enter their residency period for one-half of the fourth year of medical school with the understanding that any requirements for the M.D. degree must be met the following year. They pay a full sixteen terms of tuition and are not eligible for house staff salaries until all undergraduate requirements in the School of Medicine are discharged.

As shown in Table XXIX–6, 366 medical students were eligible to graduate between 1971 and 1974. Thirty-five, or approximately 10 percent, chose this option. This is less than the number anticipated, a response apparently influenced by three interrelated factors. The first is personal: some students were not ready to accept this level of responsibility without completing fourth-year training. The second is legal: the students were often required to have their orders and their prescriptions for patients countersigned, and some students were resentful of this arrangement. The third is pedagogical: election of an interface program of necessity committed the

Table XXIX–6. Early internship appointments by department, 1971–74

Department	1971	1972	1973	1974	Total	% Total EI
Medicine	2	3	0	2	7	20.0
Pathology	1	2	0	0	3	8.57
Pediatrics	3	5	0	1	9	25.71
Psychiatry	1	0	0	0	1	2.85
Surgery	2	5	3	5	15	42.85
Total early internship	9	15	3	8	35	
Total graduating class	80	98	91	97	366	
% each class in program	11.25	15.30	3.29	8.24	9.56	

student to an additional year at Duke, and some students felt that this commitment reduced their options for postgraduate training should they wish to leave after completion of the program.

Internship appointments by medical center

As shown in Table XXIX-7, the top ten internship selections of the classes of 1960-64 and 1970-74 were quite different, although in both periods Duke retained a significant number of her own graduates through the internship year. Military internships were less popular in the 1970's, but the fourth-place ranking of the military programs in the seventies does not indicate those government programs where postgraduate training is sponsored in a civilian medical center. There is a trend toward northeastern medical centers with Harvard and Cornell replacing Emory and Alabama in the first four institutions selected by 1970-74 graduates. Harvard hospitals, North Carolina, University of Pennsylvania, Washington University, and Utah are new among the medical centers most frequently chosen.

Internship appointments by specialty

The most popular internship appointments among the 1960-64 graduates were in medicine, in rotating internships, and in surgery. Pediatrics and mixed internships were selected less often. The 1970-74 graduates selected internships in medicine, surgery, and pediatrics most frequently. There was a significant rise in the number of graduates selecting internships in pathology

Table XXIX-7. The medical centers most frequently chosen for internships by Duke graduates, 1960-64 and 1970-74

1960-64*				1970-74			
Rank	Medical center	No.	%	Rank	Medical Center	No.	%
1	Duke University	148	37.19	1	Duke University	165	37.50
2	U.S. Military	30	7.54	2	Harvard University	18	4.09
3	Emory University	11	2.76	3	Cornell University	14	3.18
4	Alabama	10	2.51	4	U.S. Military	13	2.95
5	Med. Coll. Virginia	9	2.26	5	North Carolina	10	2.27
6	Cornell University	8	2.01	6	Univ. of Pennsylvania	9	2.05
7	Johns Hopkins	7	1.76	7	Washington University	8	1.82
8	George Washington	7	1.76	8	Johns Hopkins	7	1.59
9	Philadelphia General	7	1.76	9	University Utah	7	1.59
10	Watts Hospital	7	1.76	10	Emory University	4	0.91
	All other	141	35.69		All Other	185	42.00
	Total Graduates	398	100		Total Graduates	440	100

*Information not available on two 1960 graduates.

and psychiatry. The rotating and mixed internships were less often selected by the 1970–74 group while the new specialty of family practice began to be recognized by students as a viable career choice, as seen in Table XXIX–8.

Geographic location of graduates in practice

The greatest number of graduates of the 1960–64 classes are living in North Carolina and Florida. California and Texas also appear to have provided attractive professional opportunities for this group. Of the more recent graduates (1970–73), the greater number are in North Carolina, California, Maryland, New York, and Pennsylvania. These students, however, are still in the postgraduate phases of their medical education and their listing reflects this fact rather than where they will finally settle. Table XXIX–9 describes their distribution.

General activity of Duke graduate groups

Table XXIX–10 compares all Duke graduates, all U.S. physicians, and the two curricular groups under study with respect to their general activities in Patient Care, Teaching, Administration, and Research. The vast majority of all groups are involved in patient care activities. Within this patient care group more Duke graduates are office based than hospital based, with the exception of the 1970–73 graduate group whose major activities are involved in postgraduate training, and are therefore hospital based.

More than 15 percent of the 1960–64 graduate group is involved in teaching, administration or research, compared to 11 percent for all graduates,

Table XXIX–8. Internship appointments by specialty*

Specialty	1960–64 No.	1960–64 %	1970–74 No.	1970–74 %
Medicine	124	31.15	173	29.41
Rotating	116	29.07	24	5.47
Surgery	84	21.10	82	18.68
Pediatrics	47	11.80	65	14.80
Mixed	14	3.51	0	0
Pathology	7	1.76	31	7.06
Psychiatry	1	0.25	32	7.29
Family Practice	0†	—	16	3.64
Obstetrics—Gynecology	0†	—	1-0	2.27
Radiology	0†	—	3	0.68
Anesthesiology	1	0.25	1-	0.22
Other (Biological Sciences)	4		2	
Total	398		439	

*Information not available on two 1960 graduates and one 1974 graduate.
†Internships not offered by these specialties at this time.

Table XXIX–9. Graduates by current state of practice or training (1975)

| | 1960–64 | | | 1970–73 | |
State	Number	% Total	State	Number	% Total
North Carolina	95	24.17	North Carolina	101	31.36
Florida	43	10.94	California	23	7.14
California	30	7.63	Maryland	23	7.14
Texas	23	5.85	New York	18	5.59
Virginia	22	5.59	Pennsylvania	17	5.27
South Carolina	22	5.59	Massachusetts	14	4.34
New York	19	4.83	Texas	13	4.03
Georgia	12	3.05	Florida	12	3.72
Massachusetts	12	3.05	Ohio	11	3.41
Maryland	11	2.79	Georgia	9	2.79
Pennsylvania	11	2.79	Colorado	9	2.79
District of Columbia	10	2.54	Other U. S.	57	17.70
Other U.S.	75	19.08	FPO–APO & Unknown	15	4.65
FPO–APO & Unknown	8	2.03			
Total	393		Total	322	

Data for this table taken from Beverly C. Martin, *Medical School Alumni*. Rockville, Maryland: Aspen Systems Corporation, 1975. pp. 424–25. This source shows seven fewer doctors in the 1960–64 group and seventeen fewer in the 1970–73 group than do official Duke University records. This table and those following are based on Martin's figures. The differences are not statistically significant and are probably attributable to acceleration and deceleration of the progress of individual students.

Table XXIX–10. Duke graduates by activity and year of graduation

	All active U.S. physicians			All Duke graduates			1960–64 graduates			1970–73 graduates		
	N=366379	% Total	%	N=2761	% Total 14.23	%	N=393	% Total 14.23	%	N=322	% Total 11.66	%
Patient Care	295257	80.58		2314	83.81		320	81.42		280	86.95	
Office based	201435	54.98	68.22	1722	62.36	74.41	281	71.50	87.81	17	5.27	6.07
Hospital based	93822	25.60	31.77	592	21.44	25.58	39	9.92	12.18	263	81.67	93.92
Interns	11953	3.26	4.04	48	1.73	2.07	—	—		48	14.90	17.14
Resident	46299	12.64	15.68	317	11.48	13.69	5	1.27	1.56	190	59.00	67.85
Resident staff	35570	9.70	12.04	227	8.22	9.80	34	8.65	10.62	25	7.76	8.92
Other professional activity	29110	7.94		304	11.01		60	15.26		14	4.34	
Teaching	6183	1.68	21.24	69	2.49	22.69	21	5.34	35.00	—	—	—
Administration	11959	3.26	41.08	120	4.34	39.47	14	3.56	23.33	4	1.24	28.57
Research	8332	2.27	28.62	102	3.59	33.55	23	5.85	38.33	10	3.10	71.42
Other	2636	0.72	9.05	13	0.47	4.27	2	0.50	3.33	—	—	—
Not classified—inactive or address unknown	42012	11.46		143	5.17		13	3.30	—	28	8.69	—

Data for this table taken from Beverly C. Martin, *Medical School Alumni*. Rockville, Maryland: Aspen Systems Corporation, 1975, pp. 344.368.

Table XXIX–11. Active U.S. and Duke graduates by specialty (1975) (% of total)

Specialty	All active U.S. physicians	All active Duke physicians	U.S. physicians 1960–64	Duke physicians 1960–64	U.S. physicians 1970–73	Duke physicians 1970–73
Medical	24.06	33.71	25.98	30.27	32.95	39.13
Surgical	26.13	30.64	29.57	38.16	20.88	20.49
Other	23.13	21.76	26.26	23.91	27.09	25.46
General practice	15.85	8.69	14.20	4.32	7.92	7.14
Primary care (OB, Med, Ped)	24.83	31.87	25.62	26.71	36.51	28.57
Miscellaneous	10.08	5.17	3.99	3.30	11.14	8.69

Data for this table taken from Beveral C. Martin, *Medical School Alumni*. Rockville, Maryland: Aspen Systems Corporation, 1975. pp 122–23. 181–82.

and 7.94 percent of all active U.S. physicians. Considerably more Duke graduates indicate their participation in teaching and research activities than the national group, and this participation is even greater in the 1960 study group with 38.33 percent listing research activity.

Specialization

The relative percentages of all Duke graduates, including the 1960–64 study group, practicing some medical or surgical specialty is considerably greater than the percentages of all active U. S. physicians practicing in the same general areas (see Table XXIX–11. The number of recent graduates nationwide, and from Duke in particular, entering surgical specialties is less in the 1970's than in earlier decades, while more of the recent graduates appear to be studying in fields related to medical specialties. When sub-specialty options are selected, however, this percentage may decrease somewhat.

The percentage of Duke graduates (8.69 percent) in general practice is low in comparison to the percentage of U. S. physicians in the same area (15.85 percent). Even more impressive is the smaller percentage (4.32 percent) of the 1960 group in general practice. However, 7.14 percent of the 1970 group training in general practice compares favorably to all U. S. physicians in general practice at that time. These figures for the seventies may well be misleading because of students still in training. Another ten year period will give a more accurate picture.

The major sub-specialty areas of the groups under study are indicated in Table XXIX–12. The specialty listings do not necessarily reflect board certification; rather, they indicate the specialty as the major field of concentration designated by the physician. Duke representation in the area comprising Primary Care exceeds the national representation. Strong cardiovascular programs at Duke over the years probably account for the relatively high number of Duke graduates in this sub-specialty.

The graduate group 1960–64 is well represented in Primary Care, Internal Medicine, Pediatrics, and Ophthalmology. The percentage of 1960–64 Duke graduates in Orthopedic Surgery and Cardiovascular Diseases exceeds the percentage contemporary group of all U.S. physicians. Comparison of specialty practice area with internship selection is difficult because many (116, or 29.36 percent) of the 1960–64 graduate group selected rotating internships. In addition, the large groups (123, or 31.13 percent) interning in internal medicine and surgery (84, or 21.26 percent) are now dispersed in subspecialty areas. Only five members of the 1960–64 group interned in Pathology, while fifteen currently practice Pathology. More striking is the number of psychiatrists. While only one member entered psychiatry directly from medical school 30, or 7.63 percent of the 1960–64 graduate group, practice psychiatry.

The more recent graduate group (1970–73) is still in postgraduate training

Table XXIX–12. The graduates by subspecialty

Subspecialty	Total U.S. physicians		Total Duke physicians		U.S. physicians 1960–64		Duke 1960–64		U.S. physicians 1970–73		Duke 1970–73	
	n 286,741	%/total	n 3042	%/total	n 37,348	%/total	n 393	%	n 36,956	%	n 312	%
Primary care	71,219	24.83	880	28.92	9,569	25.62	105	26.71	13,495	36.51	92	29.48
General practice	45,471	15.85	240	7.88	5,304	14.20	17	4.32	2,928	7.92	23	7.37
Internal medicine	39,560	13.79	446	14.66	4,924	13.18	45	11.45	8,757	23.69	46	14.74
OB/GYN	16,330	5.69	170	5.58	2,429	6.50	26	6.61	1,684	4.55	10	3.20
Psychiatry	16,541	6.39	167	5.48	3,068	8.21	30	7.63	1,898	5.13	21	6.73
Pediatrics	15,329	5.57	264	8.67	2,216	5.93	34	8.65	3,054	8.35	36	11.53
General surgery	24,037	8.38	220	7.23	2,340	6.26	15	3.81	3,914	10.59	43	12.78
Radiology	12,518	4.36	121	3.97	2,114	5.66	18	4.58	1,191	3.22	7	2.24
Orthopedic surg.	9,372	3.26	109	3.58	1,695	4.53	26	6.61	806	2.18	4	1.28
Ophthalmology	9,370	3.26	117	3.84	1,600	4.28	34	8.65	630	1.70	2	0.64
Pathology	7,372	2.57	100	3.28	1,315	3.52	15	3.81	832	2.25	24	7.69
Anesthesiology	7,674	2.67	40	1.31	1,268	3.39	5	1.27	561	1.51	1	0.32
Urologic surgery	5,276	1.83	70	2.30	940	2.51	13	3.30	224	0.60	3	0.96
Cardiovascular dis.	5,026	1.75	98	3.22	973	2.60	18	4.58	13	0.03	—	

Data for this table taken from Beveral C. Martin, *Medical School Alumni*. Rockville, Maryland: Aspen Systems Corporation, 1975. pp. 122–23, 181–82.

but several career selection patterns are already evident. There is strong representation in primary care fields, internal medicine, general surgery, and pediatrics which parallels to some extent the pattern of internship selection for this group (Table XXIX–6). It is likely that the percentage of graduates currently in internal medicine and surgery will decrease as they sub-specialize. There is an apparent increase in graduates training in pediatrics and pathology. The figure for pathology may be more significant because graduates in the early 1970's tend to enter this field at the internship point.

Specialty board certification

Across the top of the columns of Table XXIX–13 are indicated the number and percentage of board-certified physicians in the U.S. and those who graduated in 1960–64 and 1970–73. It is apparent that consideration of the classes of 1970–73 is inappropriate because the majority of these graduates are in early postgraduate training and not eligible for specialty board cer-tification. Of the 1960's group 66 percent have one board, 6 percent two boards, and 28 percent have no board certification. These figures compare favorably with the corresponding figures for total U.S. physicians.

Table XXIX–13. Board certification and year of graduation (1975)

	Total U.S. Physicians		U.S. physicians classes 60–64		U.S. physicians classes 70–73	
All U.S. active schools	286,741	%	37,348	%	36,956	%
No Board	162,298	56.60	15,036	40.25	36,425	98.56
1 Board	119,608	41.71	21,501	57.56	531	1.43
2 Boards	4,813	1.67	809	2.15		
3 Boards	22	0.01	2	0.01		

	Total graduates		60–64		70–73	
Duke University	2,761	%	393	%	322	%
No Board	1,239	44.87	110	27.98	316	98.13
1 Board	1,424	51.57	260	66.15	6	1.86
2 Boards	98	3.54	23	5.85	—	
3 Boards	—		—		—	

Data for this table taken from Beverly C. Martin, *Medical School Alumni*. Rockville, Mary-land: Aspen Systems Corporation, 1975, pp. 670,676.

Duke graduates in academic medicine

The data in Tables XXIX–14a and XXIX–14b indicate that 75 members (19 percent) of the 1960–64 group of 395 Duke graduates hold academic positions on medical school faculties across the United States. Of these

Table XXIX–14a. Duke graduates (1960–64) on U.S. medical school faculties

Class of	Total	Chairman or div. head	Professor	Associate professor	Assistant professor	Other
1960	12	2	2	8	2	–
1961	18	5	1	4	11	2
1962	14	2	–	6	8	–
1963	15	5	3	4	8	–
1964	16	3	1	3	11	1
Total	75	17	7	25	40	3

Table XXIX–14b. Duke graduates (1960–64) on medical school faculties by specialty

Specialty	Chairman or div. head	Professor	Associate professor	Assistant professor	Other	Total professorial ranks
Medicine	6	3	4	17	2	26
Surgery	2		8	8		16
Pediatrics	2	2	6	6		14
Psychiatry	3	1	1	2		4
Ophthalmology			1	2	1	4
Radiology	1		1	3		4
Pathology	1		3			3
Ob–Gyn	1		1	1		2
Biochemistry	1	1				1
Family medicine				1	1	

Data for this table provided by the American Association of Medical Colleges, 1 Dupont Circle, Washington, D.C.

faculty members seventeen (23 percent) are departmental chairmen or division heads, seven are full professors, twenty-five associate professors, and forty are assistant professors. When this group of Duke graduates who are faculty members is considered by specialty field, twenty-six have appointments in medicine, sixteen in surgery, and fourteen in pediatrics. Other specialties represented include four each in psychiatry, ophthalmology, and radiology; three in pathology; two in obstetrics; one each in biochemistry and family medicine.

Conclusions

In comparing certain characteristics of medical students graduating under the traditional curriculum at Duke University (classes of 1960–64) with the students graduating under the new curriculum (classes of 1970–74) the following statements may be made:

1. *Sex and race:* Increasing the size of the medical school class has increased the number of graduates from 395 in 1960–64 to 436 for the period 1970–74.

Increasing representation of women and minority groups is apparent and continues to increase in the middle seventies.

2. *Geographic origin:* Through recruitment trips and interviews the geographic origins of the 1970–74 graduate group are broader than the 1960–64 group. There is increased representation from Middle Atlantic, North Central, New England, Pacific, and Mountain regions.

3. *National intern matching plan:* Duke graduates continue to do well in competition for postgraduate training programs. Eighty-nine percent and 81 percent of both study groups were matched to one of their three choices. There has been a decline in percentage of Duke graduates being selected for their first choice (70 percent, 1960–64; 56 percent for the 1970–74 group). Because more students move at their own pace through the medical curriculum, they are often free to make earlier arrangements for postgraduate training and may not participate in the matching plan.

The graduates of the 1970's selected different medical centers for their internships than did the 1960's group. In both groups Duke University Medical Center retained over 35 percent of her graduates for their internship year. However, Harvard, Cornell, and North Carolina received a considerable number of Duke graduates of the new curriculum.

When specialty fields are compared more graduates of the new curriculum undertook internships in internal medicine and pediatrics and slightly less in general surgery. Considerable numbers of recent graduates entered pathology and psychiatry at the internship level, and sixteen recent graduates selected training in family medicine.

4. *Current geographic location and general professional activity:* The majority of Duke medical graduates from 1960–64 practice in the southeastern region of the country, with North Carolina, Florida, Virginia, South Carolina, and Georgia being well represented. Eighty-one percent of the 1960's group are involved in patient care activities with the vast majority being office based. Fifteen percent of the 1960–64 graduate group is involved in teaching, research, and administration. Comparison with the 1970s study is not appropriate because this group is still involved in postgraduate training programs.

5. *Specialty and subspecialty:* The major broad specialties represented by both study groups and indeed all active Duke and U.S. physicians are medicine and surgery. Only 4 percent of the 1960–64 graduates are in general practice, compared to 7 percent of the 1970–73 group, who appear headed in this direction.

When each medical or surgical field is considered, 11 percent of the classes of 1960–64 specialized in internal medicine, approximately 8 percent in pediatrics and ophthalmology, with 7 percent in psychiatry. The graduates of the new curriculum are presently specializing in internal medicine (14 percent), general surgery (13 percent), pediatrics (11 percent), pathology (7 percent), and general practice (7 percent). Definite percentage increases per field for the recent graduates have occurred in general surgery, general practice, medicine, pediatrics, and pathology.

Sixty-six percent of the 1960–64 graduate group have specialty boards in one field, 6 percent in two fields, and 28 percent have no board certification. This same group is well represented on faculties of U.S. medical schools having 75 (19 percent) members holding professorial ranks. Of these faculty members 17 (23 percent) are departmental chairmen or division chiefs. Most appointments are in medicine (26), with 16 in surgery, and 14 in pediatrics.

XXX. Conclusions, and a Look Ahead

William G. Anlyan, M.D.

Forces necessary for change

The post–1966 Duke Medical curriculum restored the elective principle as a basic component of medical education in order to cope with the flood of biomedical information which developed following World War II and to provide medical students with multiple pathways through the curriculum to the diverse career opportunities which this new information created. The prewar goal of supplying students in four years with knowledge sufficient to support thirty-five future years of medical practice was abandoned in favor of more limited goals: to familiarize each student with the language of biomedicine, to provide the student with a core base of biomedical knowledge, to train the student in problem-solving as the basic approach to health and medical problems, and to imbue the student with the need for a life-long process of self-education. From its founding, Duke required its graduates to gain at least two years of experience beyond medical school before the M.D. degree was awarded. In its new curriculum the conviction that medical school is one intensive phase in an educational continuum finds final expression.

Models of change on a smaller scale suggested that change could be successful. The faculty of Western Reserve School of Medicine demonstrated in the mid–1950's that the curriculum could be rearranged from a departmental basis to a categorical, organ-oriented, interdisciplinary approach. Closer to home, the Research Training Program inaugurated at Duke in 1957 under the leadership of Drs. Handler, Stead, and Wyngaarden demonstrated that a concern to produce future medical educators, competently trained in biomedical research, could be accommodated within the existing curriculum. The challenge posed by overall curriculum revision was to create a structure capable of responding simultaneously to several such concerns, thereby allowing the form of the curriculum to remain relatively unchanged as the content of the curriculum changed to meet the goals of individual students and the needs of society at large.

In a school with a strong tradition of departmental autonomy, change was unlikely without the widest possible cooperation. In 1960, with the retirement of Dr. Wilburt C. Davison, the founding Dean of the School of Medicine, Dr. Barne Woodhall became Dean and, in the next six years, eight departmental chairmanships changed hands. This turnover made it easier to ground cooperation in new concepts, as each department defined the core of its discipline in making its contribution to "what every student receiving the M.D. degree should know." Even so, the planning process ran two years longer than anticipated. For assistance during this transition, particular credit must go to The Commonwealth Fund, the Markle Foundation, and the National Fund for Medical Education for their support of planning and evaluation, first of the Research Training Program, and later of the new curriculum itself. Innovation in medical education cannot proceed far without the major contributions of these private philanthropies.

During these same years the number and quality of the Duke faculty were significantly increased through support from multiple funding sources, and particularly from the National Institutes of Health. When the faculty first considered the need for additional resources for pump-priming and sustaining the new curriculum, the price tag amounted to well over two million dollars. Careful consideration whittled this down to approximately $150,000 per year which, after five years, could be supported by institutionally generated funds, but only given continued improvement in the quality of the faculty. Here the cooperation of private and public funding agencies with Duke was critical. To the resources of the University and the contributions of the clinical faculty through the Private Diagnostic Clinics, The Commonwealth Fund added the necessary $750,000 in initiation costs and the National Institutes of Health continued to support the work of an already excellent faculty.

In 1964, when it became my privilege to succeed Dr. Woodhall as Dean, Dr. Jane Elchlepp joined our staff with responsibility for institutional planning. Dr. Elchlepp visited other schools that had multidisciplinary teaching facilities and, with the collaboration of the chairman of the basic science departments, created the Central Teaching Laboratories. Funds from the National Institutes of Health in support of the Medical Scientist Training Program allowed construction of a model interdisciplinary laboratory which was thoroughly tested before other units were built for the remainder of the medical school class. The departments, notably physiology and pathology, also pretested the core sequences in their disciplines before the new curriculum was introduced in its totality. This step-by-step development, essential to the initial success of the new program, both reflected and solidified the cooperation of faculty and students in assessing the value of each individual change.

In the years since 1966 these resources have continued to snowball. The faculty increased in size from 204 in 1966 to 472 in 1975. The excellence of their work attracted the funds necessary to build facilities to house the programs they have devised, which are described in the earlier chapters of this book, and to support the teaching of larger medical school classes. The mix of factors necessary for change during the planning years, however, was essential for this success. The information explosion, the changing role of undergraduate medical education, faculty leadership, support from public and private agencies outside the University, prolonged attention to detail in planning, and a tradition of cooperation within the school of Medicine that was adapted to new concepts: without any one of these the curriculum revision might well have failed.

A look back

Curriculum evaluation is an inexact science, particularly when a revision occurs in a program already recognized for high quality. The shift in national priorities from research to health-care delivery, the increasing recognition that undergraduate medical education is best viewed as part of a life-long process. The economic inflation, the continuing addition of new programs within an elective system, and the impossibility of exactly measuring the attitudes of faculty and students preclude absolute generalizations about the curriculum at Duke since 1966. Our experience does indicate, however, that the undergraduate medical curriculum can be completely restructured with positive results, a question unanswered since the Flexner report. In addition, the following statements seem warranted by the evidence presented in earlier chapters.

1. The elective system provides alternative pathways through the curriculum in preparation for a multiplicity of medical careers. This benefit of restructuring is the easiest to document, given the existence of the combined degree programs and the wide variety of courses available in every department. Interestingly, as national priorities and student interests have shifted, students seem to want both more and less of this. Their shorthand for the opportunities currently available is "science and smorgasbord," an expression reflecting the desire of many for pre-defined tracks appropriate for entering careers not clearly involving research. Providing guidelines without reducing the benefits of genuine elective freedom will continue to require imaginative planning.

2. Introduction of students to the wards in their second year eliminates the sophomore slump characteristic of the traditional curriclum. Although this does not significantly change the attitudes of students toward training when measured at the end of medical school it is of major importance as each class passes through. Students and faculty alike approach their work with a more consistent enthusiasm.

3. As measured in Mini-Test scores, students entered the wards knowing as much basic medical science after one year of the elective curriculum as they did after two years under the more traditional structure. Most instructors noticed that these students were not quite as well prepared for ward duty in terms of clinical procedures, but that this initial handicap was overcome within a matter of weeks. The collective judgment of the faculty is that this is a small price to pay for the career-oriented, basic science elective opportunities of the third year.

4. The equal division of teaching time in the second year among the five clinical departments has not resulted in imbalance in clinical training. Some external observers have questioned why pediatrics, obstetrics, and psychiatry should have equal time with internal medicine or surgery, and have commented on the "political" division of the second year. However, this change was effected with the full concurrence of the medical and surgical faculties, knowing full well that in the fourth year a majority of students would return to those two departments. Politics always has some influence upon the allocation of teaching time; this combination of required and elective opportunities is a dynamic rather than static compromise.

5. Student elective choices, outside the study programs and combined degree programs, favor basic science courses closely correlated with clinical experience. Without the special programs, this tendency might well direct the curriculum from the strong emphasis upon basic science originally envisioned. In the current configuration the traditional desire of most medical students to become doctors by the shortest possible route is balanced by the clearly presented opportunity to prepare for careers in medical science and teaching. Again, this type of compromise requires constant attention to curriculum planning.

6. Under the elective curriculum, a tightly structured basic science year was accepted in order to gain maximum flexibility in the advanced science year. The significant reduction in laboratory instruction in the first year is more than compensated for by the individualized instruction in laboratory technique and research methods, much of it provided by full-time researchers and technicians, which is the core of third-year electives. All of the faculty who offer courses in the basic science core regret, from time to time, the loss of opportunity to relate additional detail to basic principles. The opportunity to work with students studying limited areas related to their career goals in depth, however, creates a level of general excitement unmatched, except on an occasional basis, within the structure of the traditional curriculum.

7. Within the Medical Center, programs that began purely as research efforts have evolved into interdisciplinary research and teaching projects. This has happened in such diverse areas as the study of aging and human development, hyperbaric medicine, and neural sciences. Similarly, courses for undergraduate medical students have been added to offerings once reserved for fellows and house staff in such areas as the study of cancer and of cardiovascular problems. Both the basic science and clinical departments have benefitted from this spinoff of research and research training into education.

8. New curriculum students exhibit somewhat greater stability in making career preference choices. Without improvement in this index, the complexities in planning an elective program in the third and fourth years would have been unmanageable. Further improvement probably can be gained best by experimenting with the relationship between the last two years of college

and the first of medical school, moving some basic medical science back into the college curriculum so that students can compare their experience in this area with other courses in the arts and sciences generally.

9. The elective curriculum has increased interchange among the School of Medicine and other components of the University. The combined degree programs are only the most obvious evidence of this development. The basic medical science departments, especially Biochemistry, Anatomy, and Microbiology, have offered their "core" courses to Trinity College undergraduates as well. Medical students in combined degree programs benefit, when they leave the Medical Center to work for the second degree, from interaction with graduate peers pursuing professional goals. The undergraduate connection may in the future allow Trinity College students to assess more accurately their chances for success in medical education. Since only about 25 percent of applicants actually enter medical school, experiments in screening will become increasingly important in the future in order that the best undergraduate students choose early fields they will be able to enter.

10. The elective curriculum is extremely expensive, both in dollars and in faculty time. Federal capitation is beginning to drop, and state capitation has remained at a constant level for the past three years. During the nine-year period 1966–75, funds from the University's endowment remained stable, although they dropped slightly last year. Fortunately, the clinical departments have largely financed their own programs, particularly by earnings contributed through the Private Diagnostic Clinics. Only this support and success in obtaining research grants have made it possible to finance the number and quality of faculty required by this curriculum structure. These factors mean that not all institutions can establish a curriculum such as has evolved at Duke. Variants might well be considered by other schools, however, knowing now that restructuring based on local conditions can achieve positive results.

A look ahead

The Duke curriculum is a drastic change from a previously successful model. A decade of experience with the curriculum has demonstrated two things: that drastic change in medical education need not dilute the quality of that education, and that elective freedom is necessary if students are to choose among the many careers open to physicians. Final evaluation of the worth of this restructuring is decades away, when the accomplishments of the current student generation are judged retrospectively. Yet provisional judgment must be passed, for, as Dr. Elchlepp has pointed out, the first order of national priorities in health affairs has changed twice since this curriculum was planned in the early 1960's. Future change promises to come with similar rapidity.

The demand uniquely placed upon medical education is that it be both conservative and experimental simultaneously. Provisional judgment of the

Duke experience, both within the profession and without, will be by this standard, although the standard will take variant forms. At Duke, the question will be whether or not the planning process continues to generate consistent enthusiasm from faculty and students. Faculty will require that the curriculum incorporate and transmit both the essence and the variety of biomedical knowledge. Students will insist that the courses and choices they confront speak both to their individual aspirations and to the needs of the society from which they come. Beyond Duke, professional peers must find that Duke graduates have indeed chosen experiences which provide advantages in solving increasingly complex problems of health care and delivery if the judgment is to be favorable.

Personal and direct professional feedback, however, will be only half the story. American society, and its health needs, change at a pace that sets its own evaluative agenda, and medical schools have neither the time nor the resources necessary to restructure to meet each social challenge. The value of the Duke curriculum to the decades immediately ahead will be as a successful structural model capable of accommodating the changes forced by future social experimentation.